N_____

Guide to

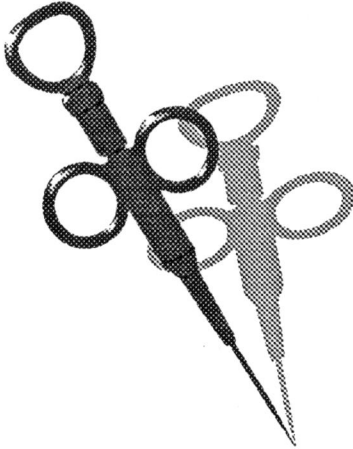

Medical Museums

in Britain

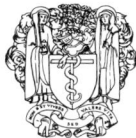

Royal Society of Medicine Services Ltd

Royal Society of Medicine Services Limited
1 Wimpole Street London W1M 8AE
150 East 58th Street New York NY 10155

British Library Cataloguing in Publication Data
A catalogue record for this book is available from the British
Library

ISBN 1-85315-206-4

Graphics & Phototypesetting by van Koetsveld Konsulting,
9 Radford House, Eden Grove, London N7 8HA
Printed in Great Britain by Henry Ling Ltd at the Dorset Press, Dorchester, Dorset

Acknowledgements

The idea for a guide book on medical history was born from my twenty year love of nursing and my subsequent training as a professional guide. To link the two interests under one title seems a logical step as no such book has hitherto been published which incorporates many of the collections of medical instruments in museums, the homes of medical men, reconstructed surgeries and pharmacies, spas or physic gardens that are open to the public in Britain.

I am grateful to Robin Price from the Wellcome Institute for encouraging me in this venture and Howard Croft from the Royal Society of Medicine who has kindly agreed to publish the book. I would also like to thank the Wellcome Trust for assisting me with a grant towards the maps and layout of the book. I am much indebted to all the curators, keepers and archivists of the museums who have given me so much valuable help and information. To all my friends in other aspects of the History of Medicine I would like to say thank you and especially to my husband Neil.

Contents

SCOTLAND

WALES

Introduction

Britain has a rich heritage of medical history. Notably the early hospitals of the eighteenth century as well as the avid collectors of the eighteenth and nineteenth centuries who have left us a rare collection of medical instruments, books and artefacts. Many doctors and pharmacists of this century have also given the tools of their trade to local museums and heritage centres.

To track down these exciting and fascinating collections that are open to the general public has given me much enjoyment over the last year. Often one discovery has led to another, and I am extremely grateful to all the curators and keepers of the many museums who have helped me. I have not included the medical and pathological museums in the medical schools and universities, as these are used primarily for teaching and are often not open to the general public. Some of the objects in the general museums, however, are held in reserve collections and can be seen 'by appointment only'. Perhaps as the interest in the history of medicine grows, and since it is part of the national curriculum linked with social history, these items will be seen on permanent display in the future. Sometimes it is difficult for the curators to identify the medical instruments and equipment and any help from medical persons would be gratefully appreciated.

I started by concentrating on medical collections held in museums - mainly instruments, prescription books, case notes and medicine containers, but soon realised that the large 'street' museums had whole buildings and shop fronts to offer. Victorian or Edwardian streets usually housed a pharmacy with carboys, leech jars, bottles, cartons and other pill making equipment. The pharmacist, who diagnosed illness and dispensed his own remedies, provided eye testing charts (with pictures not letters for the illiterate), and prescribed the spectacles too. A dental surgery was often tucked in the corner for the monthly visiting dentist. The local doctor usually had a surgery in his own home, where he could perform minor operations. He often had a small dispensary for making and dispensing his own medicines.

I found that my brief widened as I researched. I have tried to include the other aspects of medicine: true physic gardens, as opposed to the culinary herb gardens found in most country house gardens, and the healing effects of water. Water has been a source of healing since pagan times and the spa towns have played a large part in the social as well as medicinal life of Britain. Today you can either drink the water or bathe in it, without the social rituals as described by Jane Austen!

Several hospitals and operating theatres still remain. The oldest pre-anaesthesia (1846) operating theatre can be visited to-day, hidden in the roof of a church in Southwark. A hospital, specifically built by an employer for his workers, sits high on a Welsh hillside - complete with operating table and small ward with iron bedsteads. A grim reminder of the dreadful injuries which beset the slate workers while engaged in that most dangerous of work.

The houses connected with medical men and women are, I think, fascinating places to visit. Edward Jenner and his experiments with the cow-pox in Gloucestershire and Charles Darwin and his theory on the Origin of the Species, who lived at Downe in Kent. To understand how a man lived is to understand the impact of his often revolutionary views on the scientific thinking of the day.

The armed forces have given great impetus and innovation to medicine and the development of their ability to treat those on the battlefield and on the home front has been displayed in a number of museums throughout Britain. Aldershot, as the 'Home of the British Army' covers the RAMC, Nurses and Dentists, while Portsmouth's ships show the Navy in action, particularly during the Napoleonic wars. Together with the transport collections, a prisoner of war camp and German underground hospitals, a picture is created of Britain's armed medical services at work in times of hardship and war.

London has by reputation the largest number of medical history museums, libraries and places of interest. I have tried to tread a sensible path through the maze of pathology museums and small specialised collections to give only those that are most accessible. The greatest collector of all was Sir Henry Wellcome and a part of his enormous collection is well displayed at the top of the Science Museum.

There are a number of statues in the city and of course the famous 'blue plaques'. Those dedicated to the medical profession confront the ordinary passer-by with Britain's achievements in the field of medicine and are, I feel, not to be missed.

Where to end? I have not included any church plaques or burial places or the iron-clad tombs, built to frustrate the body-snatchers - they deserve another book! Neither have I included all the collections from the psychiatric hospitals, many due to close in the near future. The fate of their historic items, in many cases, is yet to be decided. Nor have I included any of the collections that are held by today's doctors in their surgeries and consulting rooms. I hope these will remain intact and identified for future generations to enjoy.

Such a small country has so much to offer the traveller in the field of medical history. Collections change as further items are donated and discovered but, with apologies to those museums I have erroneously omitted, I hope this guide will give you a taste of what is on offer and that you will have as much enjoyment in visiting as I have had in writing.

Counties

Counties of England and the Channel Islands

Name	Map Number
Avon	11
Bedfordshire	35
Berkshire	17
Buckinghamshire	26
Cambridgeshire	37
Channel Islands	63
Cheshire	31
Cleveland	51
Cornwall	1
Cumbria	49
Derbyshire	39
Devon	2
Dorset	3
Durham	52
Essex	33
Gloucestershire	19
Greater Manchester	40
Hampshire	9
Hereford & Worcestershire	20
Hertfordshire	34
Humberside	47
Kent	24
Lancashire	41
Leicestershire	38
Lincolnshire	43
London	25
Merseyside	32
Norfolk	42
Northamptonshire	27
Northumberland	54
Nottinghamshire	44
Oxfordshire	18
Shropshire	21
Somerset	4
Staffordshire	30
Suffolk	36
Surrey	16
East Sussex	23
West Sussex	15
Tyne & Wear	53
Warwickshire	28
West Midlands	29
Wiltshire	10
North Yorkshire	48
South Yorkshire	45
West Yorkshire	46

Counties of Scotland

Name	Map Number
Dumfries & Galloway	50
Lothian	57
Strathclyde	56
Tayside	60
Fife	59
Central	58
Grampian	62
Highland	61
Borders	55

Counties of Wales

Name	Map Number
Dyfed	8
Mid Glamorgan	6
South Glamorgan	5
West Glamorgan	7
Gwent	12
Gwynedd	14
Clwyd	22
Powys	13

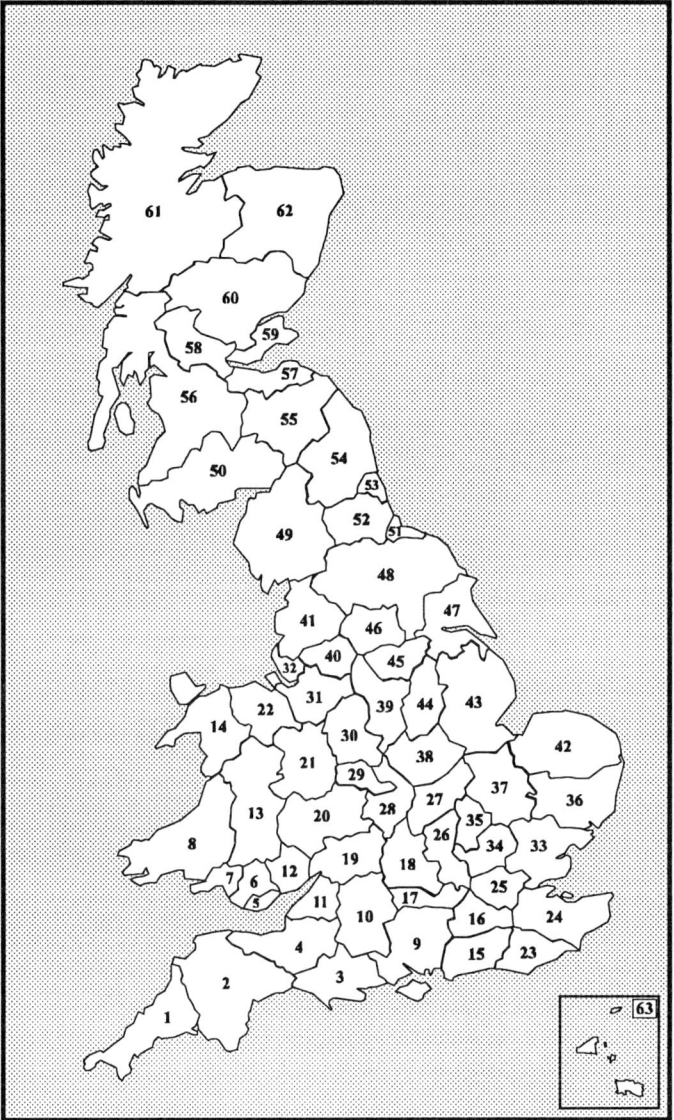

ENGLAND

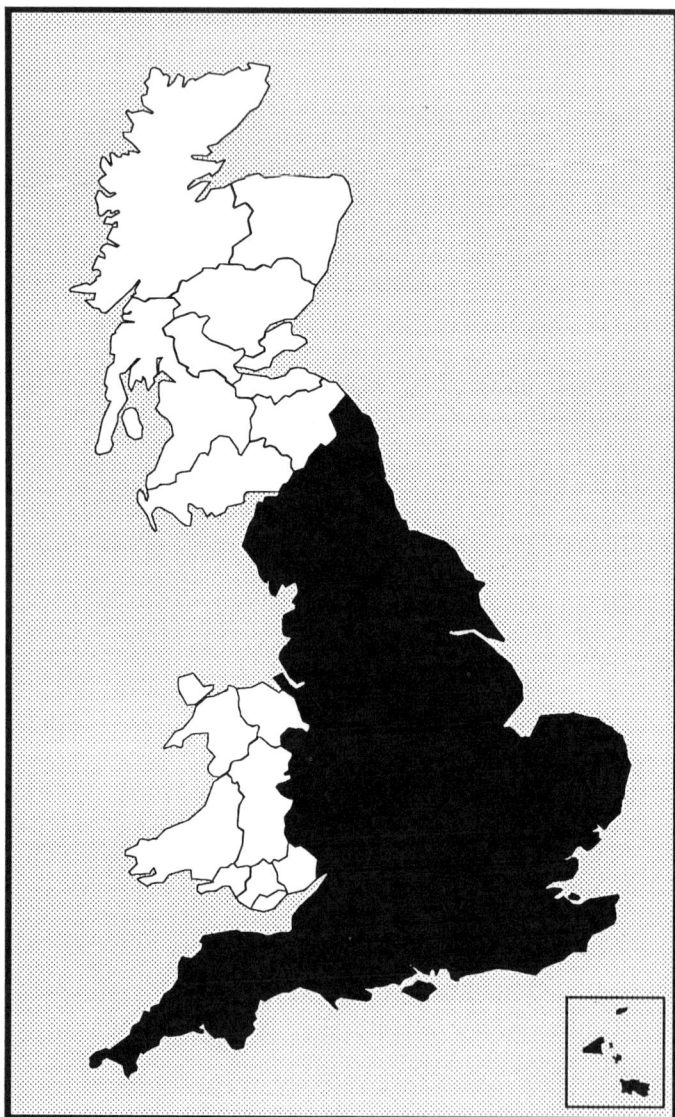

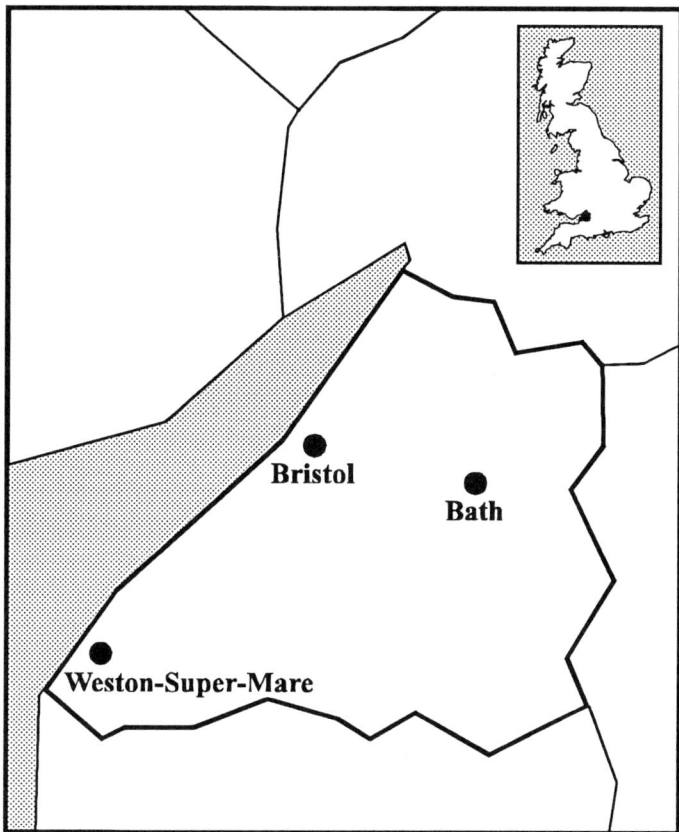

THE AMERICAN MUSEUM IN BRITAIN

CLAVERTON MANOR
BATH
AVON BA2 7BD

☎ TELEPHONE: 0225-460 503
OPEN: TUESDAY - SUNDAY .... MUSEUM: 2.00 - 5.00
                                 .... GROUNDS: 1.00 - 6.00
                  END MARCH - END OCTOBER
                  B.H. MONDAY & PRECEEDING SUNDAY ... 11.00 - 5.00
ADMISSION: CHARGE

SHOP & HERB SHOP. COUNTRY STALL. REFRESHMENTS.
TOILETS.

 ♿ DISABLED ACCESS TO GROUND FLOOR.

The elegant 19th century manor house set in superb gardens shows the development of the American way of life from the 17th to the 19th centuries. A series of furnished rooms include a Puritan keeping room of the 1680's, a tavern kitchen of the 1770's, a mid 18th century parlour and a later country-style bedroom. Shaker furniture, American Indians and some exquisite patch-work quilting are displayed in other galleries.

In the 19th century country store are a selection of medicinal glass bottles and jars. One is labelled 'Indian Cough Syrup', another 'Dr. Schenck's Tonic' and 'Glover's Imperial Mange Cure'. The patent medicines have 'Life Everlasting' herbs and 'Dr. Hardy's Magical Pain Destroyer'!

In the basement is a display of miniature rooms, made by Mr. J.H. Hoffheimerk an American business man in his spare time in 1955. Amongst them is an Apothecary's shop of 1885.

HERSCHEL HOUSE & MUSEUM

19 NEW KING STREET
BATH
AVON

☎ TELEPHONE: 0225-311 342
OPEN: MONDAY - SUNDAY ....2.00 - 5.00
ADMISSION: CHARGE
SHOP. TOILETS.

 ♿ DISABLED ACCESS DIFFCULT.

In March 1781 from the garden of this small terraced house William Herschel discovered the planet Uranus, thereby doubling the size of the known solar system.

A Hanoverian by birth he came to England and obtained the position of organist at the Octagon Chapel in Bath. An expert musician he became fascinated by astronomy and began to make his own telescopes. King George III gave him an official pension which enabled him to give up music as a career and devote his whole life to astronomy, where he was able to observe and map the star-system. He lived in Bath with his sister Caroline and the house has been turned into a museum with a replica of his telescope and other instruments. Upstairs is a tribute to his musical genius and family portraits.

In the basement is a kitchen of 1781, William's workshop where he made his specular metal mirrors and outside a small garden containing herbs and physic plants. Amongst these is angelica for a sore throat, balm for use as an antispetic, comfrey for bleeding, lovage for boils, marigold for fever, rue for indigestion, sorrel to be used to bandage sores and valarian for headaches. John Herschel, his son, went to South Africa to collect plants.

ROMAN BATHS & MUSEUM

> PUMP ROOM
> BATH
> AVON

ℭ TELEPHONE: 0225-461 111
   OPEN: MONDAY - SUNDAY ....9.00 - 5.00
   ADMISSION: CHARGE
   SHOP. REFRESHMENTS. TOILETS.
ᕦ DISABLED ACCESS TO GROUND FLOOR ONLY.

The Romans named the town Aquae Sulis between the 1st and 5th centuries and built the Great Bath and temples around the natural hot springs that rise from the ground at a constant 46.5°C, as a place of rest and relaxation for their noblemen and legionaires. The Baths fell into ruins until the Georgian era when bathing again became fashionable and Beau Nash instituted the strict social programme of 'taking the waters'. In 1741 The Royal Mineral Water Hospital for Rheumatic Diseases was founded to relieve those suffering from rheumatism, but the Roman origins are not far away and an excavated Roman pavement is on display in the basement.

To-day both the Roman Baths, the source of the thermal water and the Georgian bath can be seen on an excellent conducted tour, with an opportunity to sample the water and Bath buns in the Pump Room afterwards.

Near the Tourist Information Centre is the smaller healing spring of the Cross Bath, a place of relaxation, peace and tranquillity. Run by volunteers, open on Friday, Saturday and Sunday (mostly in the afternoon), it is hoped to restore, renovate and re-open the bath for bathing in the not too distant future.

GLENSIDE HOSPITAL

BLACKBERRY HILL
STAPLETON
BRISTOL
AVON BS16 1DD

☎ TELEPHONE: 0272-653 285 EXT. 206
OPEN: FRIDAY (WHEN POSSIBLE) ....2.00 - 4.00
ADMSSION: FREE

♿ DISABLED ACCESS - RING FIRST.

🚶 GROUPS BY ARRANGEMENT TO DR. EARLY 0454-312 929.

Bristol has led the country in the provision of services in the public sector, from the 1696 Bristol Poor Act which aimed to have one building for the destitute and homeless, orphans and idiots, with a ward for lunatics, until 1861 when the first public hospital to provide treatment for the mentally ill was founded.

Overcrowding, the Lunatics Act of 1845 and cumulative pressures had compelled the Corporation of Bristol to build a new asylum, and so on 27th February 1861 it opened; after several name changes it became known as Glenside Hospital in 1959.

In 1914 it was taken over by the War Office to become the Beaufort War Hospital and one noteable and humble member of staff was the artist Stanley Spencer, whose later paintings placed on record the day-to-day activities of the hospital. After 125 busy years the hospital is about to close and the future of the museum is far from certain.

The fascinating collection of artefacts ranges from low beds with strong gingham sheets, to china bedpans and hot water bottles, telephones and typewriters, floor polishers, cooking utensils, photographic records and the leather-bound attendants and servants register of 1897. Some of the museum is housed in a gallery overlooking the large dining hall and there keys, webbed pronged forks, a 1940's operating table, 1930's dictaphone, 1940's ECT machine, canvas straight-jackets and trousers, early fleams and syringes, medicine bottles, scales, and work by the in-patients provide a glimpse into the life of a large and busy hospital. The drawings by a schizophrenic patient in 1930 are very moving as is the chain painstakingly carved from a single piece of wood.

MONICA BRITTON EXHIBITION HALL OF MEDICAL HISTORY

FRENCHAY HOSPITAL
BRISTOL
AVON BS16 1LE

① TELEPHONE: 0272-701 212 EXT. 2626/2636
OPEN: MONDAY - FRIDAY ....9.30 - 4.30
PLEASE CONFIRM AVAILABILITY BY PHONE.
OPEN AT OTHER TIMES BY ARRANGEMENT.
PHONE DR. J.A.BENNETT ON 0272-701 212
EXT. 2262 or DR LUSH ON 0454-41212
ADMISSION: FREE

🕺 SPECIAL EXHIBITIONS. LECTURES/SEMINARS FOR
SPECIALIST GROUPS BY ARRANGEMENT. GROUP VISITS
AND FEES BY NEGOCIATION.

Originally a private house with 70 acres of land, the 18th century manor house was thought in 1913, to be the perfect setting for a children's sanatorium for TB of the bone, joints and chest. At the start of the Second World War an emergency hospital was added to Frenchay Park Sanatorium to house those who may be wounded in the air-raids. In the event the hospital beds were not needed so in May 1942, when the first American military personnel arrived, they were handed over the hospital for their own use. In 1948 it became a District General Hospital and since been a centre of excellence for West England.

Monica Britton was the wife of a local industrialist and philanthropist and on her death in 1983 her husband wanted a useful permanent memorial that would be a living and dynamic reflection of her own active life. So the Exhibition Hall, attached to the postgraduate centre at Frenchay Hospital came into being. It is run by enthusiastic doctors, with additional voluntary help, and is used for many hospital meetings and events.

The excellent display includes a 1913 dental X-ray machine, foot pedal, dental drill, 1950's suction machine, a display of the development of transurethral prostatectomy with photographs and instruments, medical sterilisers, collections of pharmacy labels and pill-making equipment including some Victorian bottles with their original contents. Assorted stethoscopes, amputation instruments, homeopathic medicine in Bristol, obstetric forceps, resuscitation and ophthalmic equipment are also shown.

WOODSPRING MUSEUM

BURLINGTON STREET
WESTON-SUPER-MARE
AVON

ⓓ TELEPHONE: 0934-621 028
OPEN: TUESDAY - SUNDAY .... 10.00 - 5.00
ADMISSION: FREE
SHOP. REFRESHMENTS. TOILETS.

♿ DISABLED ACCESS TO GROUND FLOOR.

🚶 GROUPS BY ARRANGEMENT.

Set around a tree-lined courtyard the old Gaslight Company's workshops are now home to a museum of local life. Displays of natural history, with the newest audio-visual night scene showing birds and animals of the night, a Victorian seaside holiday, mining, dairying, costumes and cameras. The pharmacy has items mostly from one shop which closed in the early 1960's. Upstairs is a reconstructed dental surgery with chair and foot pedal drill.

Next door Clara's Cottage is a seaside lodging house of the 1900's with the Nisbet collection of costume dolls in the upper rooms.

Bedfordshire

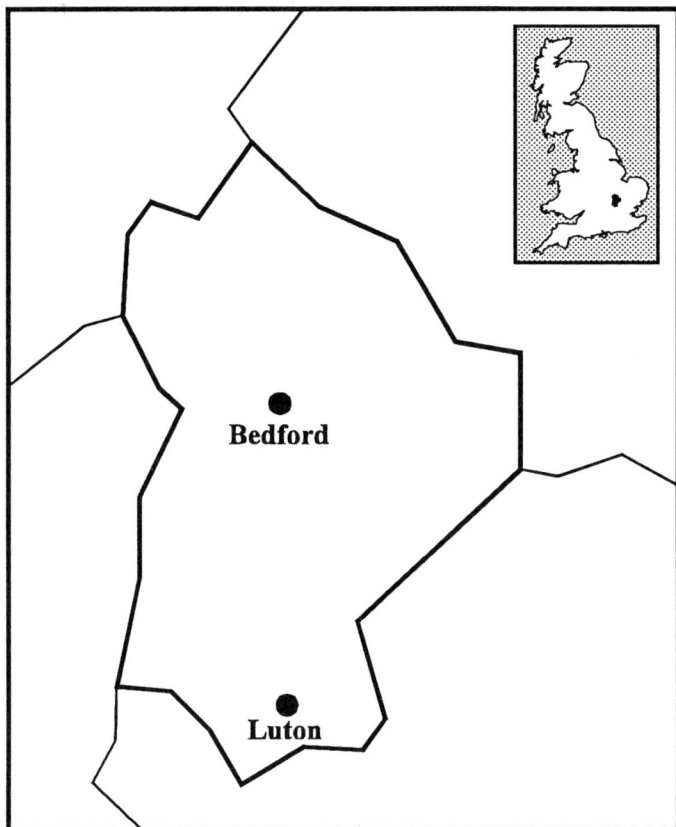

BEDFORD MUSEUM

CASTLE LANE
BEDFORD
BEDFORDSHIRE MK40 3XD

☾ TELEPHONE: 0234-353 323
OPEN: TUESDAY - SATRURDAY.............................11.00 - 5.00
         SUNDAY & B.H. MONDAYS............................2.00 - 5.00
ADMISSION: FREE
SHOP.TOILETS.

♿ DISABLED ACCESS TO ALL THE MUSEUM.

The old Higgins Castle Brewery and later clothing factory and GPO sorting office is now home to this museum of local life. Tracing the history of the people of Bedfordshire from the ice age to the 19th century there is much archeological material, local industries such as lace making and straw plaiting and domestic and agricultural bygones. In the social history displays are some items from an apothecary's shop of the 19th century including a pill board, horn scoop for medicine ingredients, a boxwood pestle and mortar, drug cabinet with a range of drugs, weighing measuring and mixing equipment and Bischof's water filter. An electric shock machine and various blood-letting equipment such as a scalpel, spring-operated scarifier, leech jar and leech applicator tubes. Dental equipment from the late 19th century includes extraction hooks and levers, a hand-drill, scalers and polished metal mirrors with some false teeth made for the Great Exhibition of 1851 from animal bone and porcelain. There is also another set on show in the geology display to demonstrate an early economic use of gold to make the plates for a set of porcelain teeth.

Bedford was the home from 1773-1790 of John Howard, the prison reformer, whose efforts led to the passing of two Acts of Parliament in 1774 providing for fixed salaries for jailers and enforcing cleanliness and elementary sanitation in the prisons. Some material is on loan from the Trustees of the Howard Reform Church.

LUTON MUSEUM & ART GALLERY

WARDOWN PARK
LUTON
BEDFORDSHIRE LU2 7HA

☎ TELEPHONE: 0582-36941
OPEN: MONDAY - SATURDAY .... 10.00 - 5.00
         SUNDAY .... 1.00 - 5.00
ADMISSION: FREE
SHOP. REFRESHMENTS. TOILETS.

♿ DISABLED ACCESS.

👫 GROUPS BY APPOINTMENT.

The magnificent park and mansion provide a suitable setting for a museum of local history and industry. A lace maker's cottage, street scene, straw plaiting and the straw hat industry, china, furniture and costumes and archaeology show the life and work of the people of Luton.

A reserve collection of medical items on loan from the Luton and Dunstable Hospital including nursing equipment, fleams, cupping sets, tooth key and an ear trumpet can be seen on application to the Keeper of Social History.

Berkshire

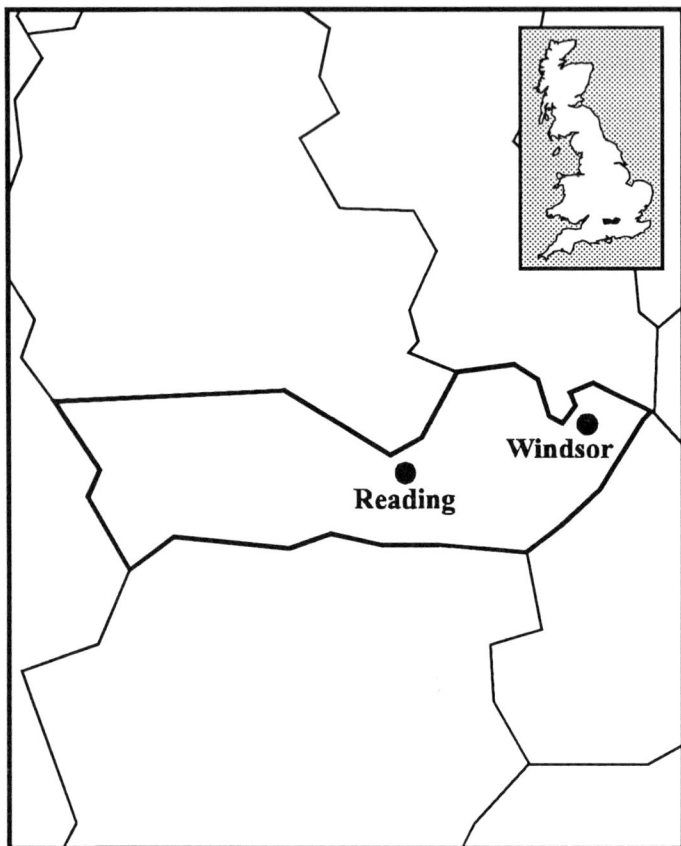

BLAKE'S LOCK MUSEUM

GASWORKS ROAD
OFF KENAVON ROAD
READING
BERKSHIRE

℡ TELEPHONE: 0734-590 630
    OPEN: MONDAY - FRIDAY ....10.00 - 5.00
                 SATURDAY & SUNDAY ....2.00 - 5.00
    ADMISSION: CHARGE
    SHOP.
♿ DISABLED ACCESS.

Housed in the Old Gasworks the museum shows the industrial and commercial life of Reading and the development of the waterways for cargo carrying and pleasure. A Victorian chemist's shop has bottles, jars, a drug run and a pill making machine.

KEELER LIMITED

CLEWER HILL ROAD
WINDSOR
BERKSHIRE SL4 4AA

☎ TELEPHONE; 0753-857 177
OPEN: BY APPONTMENT ONLY FOR SERIOUS RE-
            SEARCHERS.

The company produces opthalmic equipment and has a collection that dates from the mid 1920's. It is open only to serious researchers who should apply to the Chairman.

Buckinghamshire

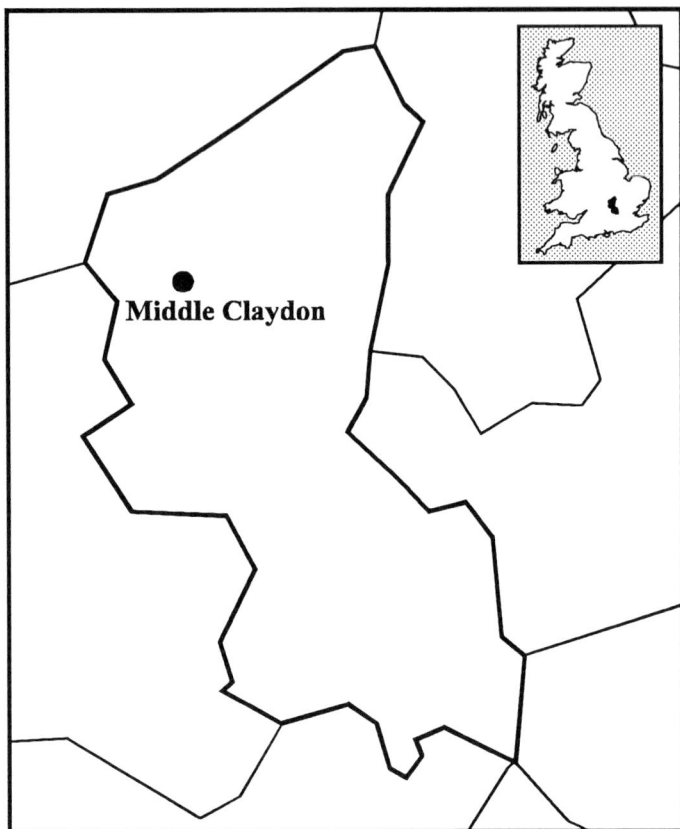

CLAYDON HOUSE

MIDDLE CLAYDON
NR. BUCKINGHAM
BUCKINGHAMSHIRE MK18 2EY

TELEPHONE: 0296-730 349
OPEN: SATURDAY - WEDNESDAY .... 1.00 - 5.00
              & B.H. MONDAY LAST ADMISSION 4.30
              IST APRIL TO END OCTOBER
ADMISSION: CHARGE, NATIONAL TRUST

REFRESHMENTS. TOILETS. ORGANIC SHOP FOR GARDEN PRODUCE AND PLANTS.

 ♿ DISABLED ACCESS TO GROUND FLOOR AND GARDENS.

 ♯ GUIDED TOURS FOR VISUALLY HANDICAPPED BY ARRANGEMENT.

The stone-faced West wing is all that remains of the ambitious house built by Ralph, Lord Verney in 1769. The brick East wing, remodelled from the early Tudor manor house, is now the home of the 5th Baronet, Sir Ralph Verney and his wife. The fine interiors with their superb wood carvings are probably the work of the mysterious and eccentric carver and cabinet-maker, Luke Lightfoot.

In 1858 Parthenope Nightingale married Sir Harry Verney. Her sister Florence spent many summers at Claydon; there is a portrait bust of her in the library, and portraits and photographs in her bedroom. In the upper lobby is a small museum with a miscellany of objects including letters from F.N., notes from her journal, a letter from Queen Victoria dated 1855, photographs, notes on nursing and mementoes from the Boer War. The Wellcome Institute has copies of all the letters from F.N. held at Claydon and a catalogue of all her letters in other locations.

Sir Harry Verney and his wife Parthenope are commemorated in the 700 year old church which stands just a few yards from Claydon House.

Florence is buried in the small country church of St. Margaret's, East Wellow, Hampshire.

Cambridgeshire

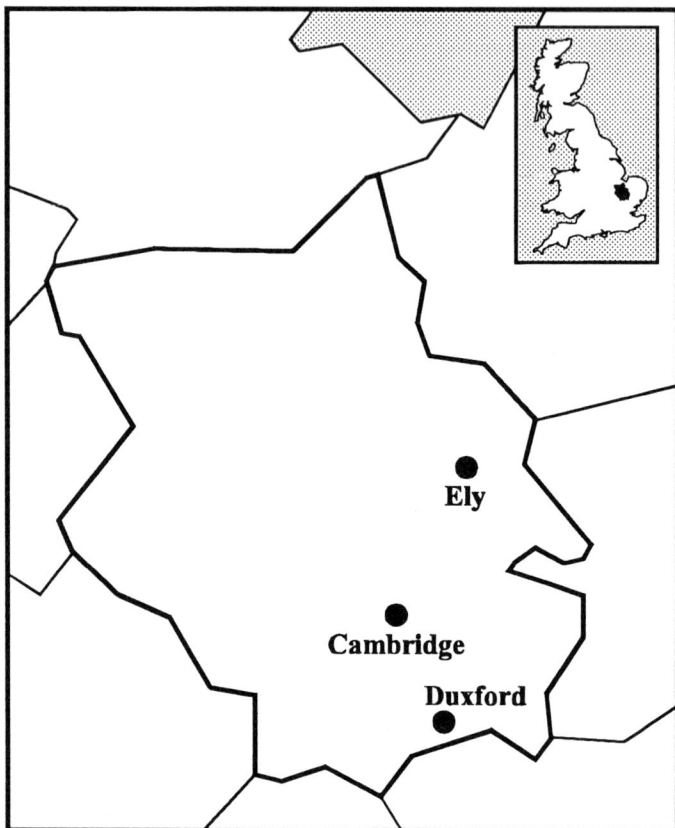

CAMBRIDGE & COUNTY FOLK MUSEUM

2-3 CASTLE STREET
CAMBRIDGE
CAMBRIDGESHIRE CB3 0AQ

TELEPHONE: 0223-355 159
OPEN: TUESDAY - SATURDAY .... 10.30 - 5.00
            SUNDAY .... 2.00 - 5.00
            OCTOBER - MARCH
            MONDAY - SATURDAY .... 10.30 - 5.00
            SUNDAY .... 2.00 - 5.00
            APRIL - SEPTEMBER
ADMISSION: CHARGE

SHOP. SPECIAL EVENTS. HOLIDAY WORKSHOPS FOR
CHILDREN & ACTIVITY DAYS.

 ♿ DISABLED ACCESS TO GROUND FLOOR.

The museum is housed in a superb 16th century building near the River Cam. It is one of the oldest private dwellings in Cambridge and for 300 years was a working inn, known as the White Horse Inn. Reminders of its colourful past can still be seen in the museum together with domestic and agricultural objects, pictures and toys all showing the rural life of the community. The medical items include drug jars, ointment pots, (one advert showing 'The Cambridge Six Hours Ointment'), Keating's cough lozenges in a metal tin, a caustic pencil, a Boots nasal and ear syringe, ceramic pestle and mortar, travelling medicine bottles and measures of the 19th century, apothecary's scales, an inhaler, mercury phials and a hydrometer, a flexible monaural stethoscope, a 19th century glass syringe with ivory plunger and boxwood case, a brass syringe of 1875, scarifier and a chemist's prescription book of 1852.

WHIPPLE MUSEUM OF THE HISTORY OF SCIENCE

FREE SCHOOL LANE
CAMBRIDGE
CAMBRIDGESHIRE CB2 3RH

♲ TELEPHONE: 0223-358 381
  OPEN: MONDAY - FRIDAY ....2.00 - 4.00
      OCCASIONALLY CLOSED IN VACATIONS
  ADMISSION: FREE
  SHOP.

 ♿ NO DISABLED ACCESS.

Housed in the historic Free School, erected in 1618 under the will of Stephen Perse of Caius College, the museum was established in 1944 when Mr. R.S. Whipple, former chairman of the Cambridge Scientific Instrument Company, presented his extensive collection of early scientific instruments and antiquarian books to the University. To this core collection have been added a great many historic instruments and over the last decade some

1,500 new items have been aquired. Included in the scientific instruments is Nairne's patent medico-electrical machine of 1785, and an electrocardiograph of 1923.

DUXFORD AIRFIELD

DUXFORD
CAMBRIDGE
CAMBRIDGESHIRE CB2 4QR

TELEPHONE: 0223-835 000
OPEN: MONDAY - SUNDAY .... 10.00 - 6.00
MID MARCH - END OCTOBER
MONDAY - SUNDAY .... 10.00 - 4.00
IST NOVEMBER-MID MARCH
ADMISSION: CHARGE
SHOP. REFRESHMENTS. TOILETS. EDUCATIONAL
PROGRAMME.

DISABLED ACCESS.

GROUPS BY ARRANGEMENT.

As part of the Imperial War Museum, Duxford's collections include military aircraft and vehicles, tanks, guns and naval exhibits and a large collection of British civil airlines. With an operational runway there are flying displays and demonstrations.

The aerodrome was built during the First World War and was one of the earliest Royal Air Force stations. It has also been home to American airmen since 1918.

Included in the static displays are two ambulances, one a Nash Ambassador Saloon converted by the Bata shoe company at its east London factory in 1940. It is typical of the wartime conversions of civil vehicles for military or civil defence use. The other is a standard Austin K2 ambulance used until the 1950's, complete with stretchers, first aid equipment, bandages etc.. Other equipment is held in store and is available by appointment; please ring the department of exhibits, Imperial War Museum on 071-416 5000.

ELY MUSEUM

28C HIGH STREET
ELY
CAMBRIDGESHIRE CB7 4HL

ⓓ TELEPHONE: 0353-666 655
OPEN: TUESDAY - SATURDAY ....10.30 - 1.00 & 2.15 - 5.00
                 SUNDAY..2.15 - 5.00
                 AND IN AUGUST...10.30 - 1.00
ADMISSION: CHARGE

♿ DISABLED ACCESS DIFFCULT AS MUSEUM IS UP-STAIRS.

A local museum devoted to the life and work of the people of Ely with collections of archeology, farm and craft utensils and the bicycle that won the world's first bicycle race. The medical items include the case of instruments used by Staff Surgeon H.S. Saunders of the Cambridgeshire Regiment in the last century with a number of saws, knives, scalpels, syringes and other equipment. A small field dressing pack, dated February 1942, was found in Ely RAF Hospital, complete with directions for use.

Channel Islands

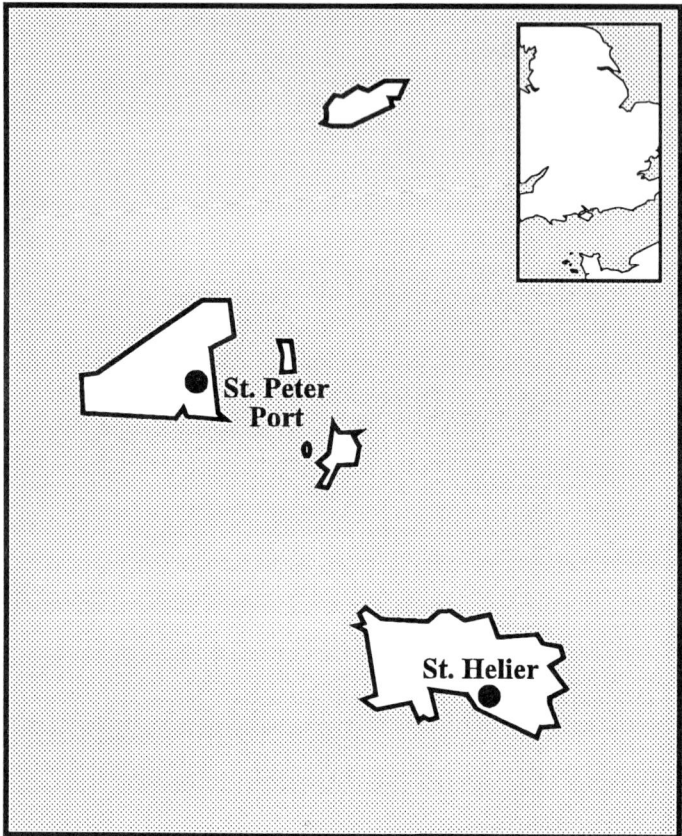

GERMAN MILITARY UNDERGROUND MUSEUM

LA VASSALERIE
ST. ANDREW'S
GUERNSEY
CHANNEL ISLANDS

☽ TELEPHONE: 0481-38205
   OPEN: MONDAY - SUNDAY
            JUNE...................................... 10.00 - 12.00 & 2.00 - 4.00
            JULY, AUGUST .... 10.00 - 12.00 & 2.00 - 5.00
            SEPTEMBER........................ 10.00 - 12.00 & 2.00 - 4.00
            OCTOBER ....2.00 - 4.00

THURDSAY & SUNDAY
NOVEMBER...2.00 - 3.00

This large underground complex of hospital and ammunition store was built by the Germans with forced labour from Europe, after they had landed in the Channel Islands in 1940. Designed to accommodate 500 patients, it could in an emergency have housed three or four times that number. The hospital was used for only 6 weeks, so at the end of the war the large items of medical equipment were removed and taken to the mainland. To-day 1 1/4 miles of corridor can be visited and much of the central heating plant and signs of the cooking arrangements can be seen. The beds remain and some small surgical instruments together with relics of the Occupation including newspapers and photographs. The scale of the tunnels and the immense amount of hard work that made them possible are a unique and grim reminder of life under the Occupation.

THE GERMAN UNDERGROUND HOSPITAL

MEADOWBANK
ST LAWRENCE
JERSEY
CHANNEL ISLANDS

☎ TELEPHONE: 0534-36493/35253
OPEN: DAILY ....9.30 - 5.30
          (WINTER TIMES VARY)
ADMISSION: CHARGE
TOILETS. SHOP.

On July 1st 1940, German airborne forces occupied the Channel Islands, their first foothold on British soil. Work on the tunnels, to be used as a barracks and ammunition store, was commenced in October 1941 and abandoned, unfinished in January 1944. The work had been carried out by skilled German civilian artisans supported by as many as 5,000 forced labourers who had been marched across Europe from Russia, Poland and France. They created an amazing construction of more than a mile of corridors hewn from the solid rock, immune to attack by land or from the air. The whole complex was converted to a hospital in January 1944. This construction, which incorporated wards for up to 500 casualities, a fully functioning operating theatre, doctors and nurses quarters and a mortuary, has been recreated with chilling realism and is one of the most comprehensive museums on the Occupation in the Channel Islands. Rare wartime archive film has been incorporated into a unique and continuous video presentation, together with photographs, letters and documents.

Cheshire

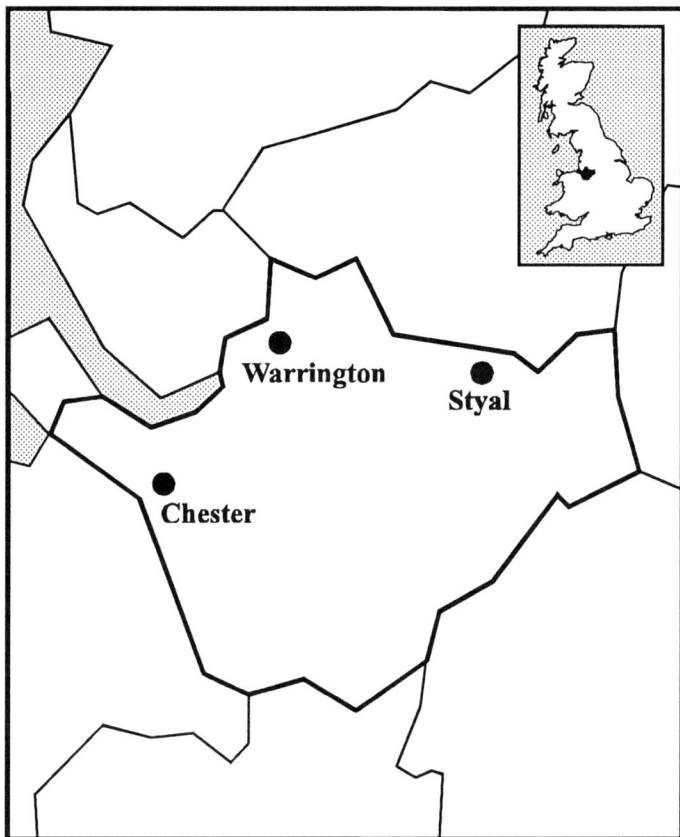

CHESTER VISITOR CENTRE

VICARS LANE
CHESTER
CHESHIRE CH1 1QX

☽ TELEPHONE: 0244-318 916
OPEN: MONDAY - SUNDAY ....9.00 - 9.00
NOVEMBER - MARCH ....9.00 - 7.00
ADMISSION: FREE
SHOP. REFRESHMENTS. TOILETS.

♿ DISABLED ACCESS.

This unusual visitor's centre is just outside the city walls and has upstairs a re-constructed Victorian street scene. Amongst the grocer's, draper's and haberdasher's is a chemist. The mahogany drug run has the usual bottles, jars, pills and potions, pill making equipment, pestle and mortar, dispensing area and many patent medicines.

There are models of Roman and Victorian Chester and a video on the history of the city.

QUARRY BANK MILL

STYAL
WILMSLOW
CHESHIRE SK9 4LA

① TELEPHONE: 0625-527 468
MILL:
OPEN: DAILY .... 11.00 - 5.00
         APRIL - END SEPTEMBER
         TUESDAY - SUNDAY .... 11.0 - 4.00
         OCTOBER - MARCH
APPRENTICE HOUSE & GARDEN:
OPEN: AS MILL IN SCHOOL HOLIDAYS
         TUESDAY .... 2.00 - 4.00
         JANUARY - APRIL,
         LATE APRIL - JULY,
         SEPTEMBER - DECEMBER
ADMISSION: CHARGE, NATIONAL TRUST
TOILETS. REFRESHMENTS. SHOP.

& DISABLED ACCESS TO PART OF INTERIOR USING STEP LIFT.

♦ ADVANCE BOOKING FOR ALL PARTIES.

A major Georgian cotton mill restored as a working museum of the cotton industry is now running again under waterpower. Set in rural parkland with a working water wheel, cloth is still produced on the historic looms and is for sale in the shop. The Apprentice house recreates life as lived by the pauper children in the 1830's with a the fascinating garden of fruit, vegetable and herbs. The owners of the Mill, the Greg family, were pioneers in providing medical services for their employees. They provided loans to establish a dispensary, a Sick Club and a Female Society, to assist with the problems of childbirth. The prescription books and other medical notebooks of Dr. Peter Holland of Knutsford still exist (1804-1827). They are kept in the archives of Manchester Central Reference Library but the Mill hope in the future to publish transcripts of Dr. Holland's note books together with a commentary. The staff at the Apprentice House are trained to interpret the notebooks and further explanatory panels on housing, enviroment, diet and working conditions are in the Mill.

MUSEUM & ART GALLERY

BOLD STREET
WARRINGTON
CHESHIRE WA1 1JG

☉ TELEPHONE: 0925-444 400/30550
OPEN: MONDAY - FRIDAY ....10.00 - 5.30
             SATURDAY ....10.00 - 5.00
ADMISSION: FREE
SMALL BOOKSTALL. (NEW SHOP & REFRESHMENTS POSSIBLY IN 1993). TOILETS.

♿ DISABLED ACCESS TO TWO FLOORS, RING FIRST.

With a large collection of natural history, geology and Egyptology and local history from Roman to medieval times this museum has a wide range of exhibits including glass, pottery, porcelain and clocks and an archive collection of photographs. A wooden stethoscope is described as one of Laennec's original instruments and is shown with three pocket microscopes, the earliest of which is reputed to be 1730.

A reserve collection has mainly 20th century instruments, donated by retired practitioners and the local hospital amongst which is a magneto-electric machine of 1880-90, an apothecary's box, a blood circulator of 1905, elbow, leg and foot splints of 1946-8 and a nasal speculum of 1904. These are available to view by appointment.

Cleveland

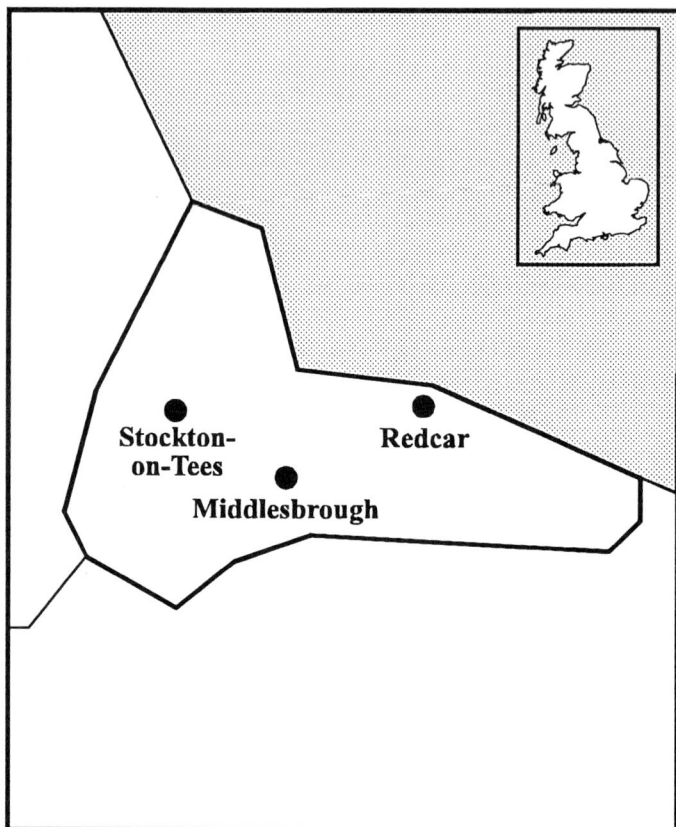

DORMAN MUSEUM

LINTHORPE ROAD
MIDDLESBOROUGH
CLEVELAND

TELEPHONE: 0642-813 781
OPEN: TUESDAY - SATURDAY ....10.00 - 6.00
ADMISSION: FREE
SHOP. TOILETS.

DISABLED ACCESS TO MAIN EXHIBITS ON GROUND FLOOR,
RING FIRST.

Opened in 1904 in memory of Lt. G.L. Dorman, who was killed in the Boer War, the museum has a fascinating collection of natural history exhibits including fossils, dinosaurs, tropical fish, an observer bee-hive and many stuffed birds, eggs and shells. A display on the history of Middlesbrough includes some medical equipment with amputation instruments and a pathology kit from the 19th century.

There is a gallery of changing exhibitions, one of which was on 'Good Health.'

KIRKLEATHAM OLD HALL MUSEUM

KIRKLEATHAM
REDCAR
CLEVELAND TS10 5NW

☎ TELEPHONE: 0642-479 500
OPEN: MONDAY - SUNDAY
                APRIL - SEPTEMBER ....9.00 - 5.00
                OCTOBER - MARCH....................................10.00 - 4.00
ADMISSION: FREE
TOILETS. REFRESHMENTS. SHOP. CHILDREN'S PLAY AREA. PICNIC AREA.

♿ DISABLED ACCESS TO GROUND FLOOR ONLY.

🚶 GROUPS BY APPOINTMENT.

Sir William Turner, born in Kirkleatham, made his fortune in London as a successful wool merchant. As Lord Mayor in 1669 he was actively involved in the rebuilding of the City after the Great Fire of 1666. His support of the poor in London through his charitable works as President of the Bridewell and Bethlem Hospitals was extended to Kirkleatham when, in 1676, he founded and endowed Sir William Turner's Hospital. It provided homes for 10 poor men and 10 women and 20 orphans, who were given a free education. To-day the Hospital still provides homes for 20 elderly men and women. In his will Sir William left money to endow a Free School for poor boys, which survived until 1738 when it became a public library and museum, poor house and in the 1840's a private home. (One occupant, Frances Jaques, attended the same nurse training school as Florence Nightingale in Kaiserworth and inspired the cottage hospital movement, founding one of the first in Middlesborough). To-day the museum depicts the lives of local people with displays on farming, trades, crafts, industires, domestic life, childhood, fashion, transport and maritime history.

There is a collection of late 19th and early 20th pharmacy equipment from Fairbanks & Franks, a Guisborough chemist. The old day-books of the William Turner Hospital can be viewed by appointment.

GREEN DRAGON MUSEUM

THEATRE YARD
STOCKTON-ON-TEES
CLEVELAND TS18 1AT

☎ TELEPHONE: 0642-674 308
OPEN: MONDAY - SATURDAY .... 9.00 - 5.00
ADMISSION: CHARGE
SHOP. TOILETS. REFRESHMENTS ACROSS THE YARD.
TOURIST INFORMATION CENTRE ATTACHED TO MUSEUM.

♿ DISABLED ACCESS TO GROUND FLOOR ONLY.

Named after possibly the oldest pub in Stockton the museum portrays the story of the famous Stockton and Darlington railway with a fascinating audio-visual presentation. Other people of Stockton have left their mark, notably Thomas Sheraton, designer and maker of fine furniture, and Dr. John Walker, inventor of the first friction match in 1827, surgeon and chemist. He called the device 'Congreves' (alluding to Congreve's rocket), later named lucifers and then matches. There is also a display on Dr. McGonigal, sanitary inspector in the 1920's and 1930's concerned with slum clearance, poverty and the high incidence of malnutrtion. A video will soon be available on his work.

There is a display on the work of the St. John's Ambulance with uniforms and equipment. Other aspects of local history can be researched in the local studies room with access to archive material.

Further exhibitions on local public health show the 18th century clean water system and links with other health material. It is hoped to show an original chemist's shop in 1993.

PRESTON PARK MUSEUM

YARM ROAD
STOCKTON-ON-TEES
CLEVELAND

☏ TELEPHONE: 0642-781 184
OPEN: MONDAY - SATURDAY....................................9.30 - 5.30
         SUNDAY..2.00 - 5.30
ADMISSION: FREE
TOILETS. PARKING. REFRESHMENTS. PICNIC AREA.

♿ DISABLED ACCESS TO GROUND FLOOR.

Originally built in 1825, Colonel Sir Robert Ropner, a local shipbuilder enlarged and modernised the hall in the late 1800's and after a period of vaccancy it was aquired by Stockton Borough Council who opened it as a museum in 1953. Housing the bequest of paintings of Miss Anne Clepham, including Georges de la Tour's Dice Players and the Spence bequest of arms, armour and 'objects de vertu', the museum has a strong Victorian flavour, including the costume and toy gallery, domestic bygones and recreated period rooms. The period street includes a grocer, tobacconist, draper, pawnbroker, ironmonger, bookshop and chemist. This late Victorian shop came from Richmond, Yorkshire, and shows the mahogany fittings, glass jars, apothecary's scales and drug register. The museum is trying to keep alive traditional skills and a farrier, blacksmith and wood worker may sometimes be seen demonstrating their expertise. The Museum stands in over a 100 acres of parkland with riverside walks, children's play area and a historical walk along part of the orginal Stockton to Darlington railway trackbed, the world's first railway built for passenger travel.

Cornwall

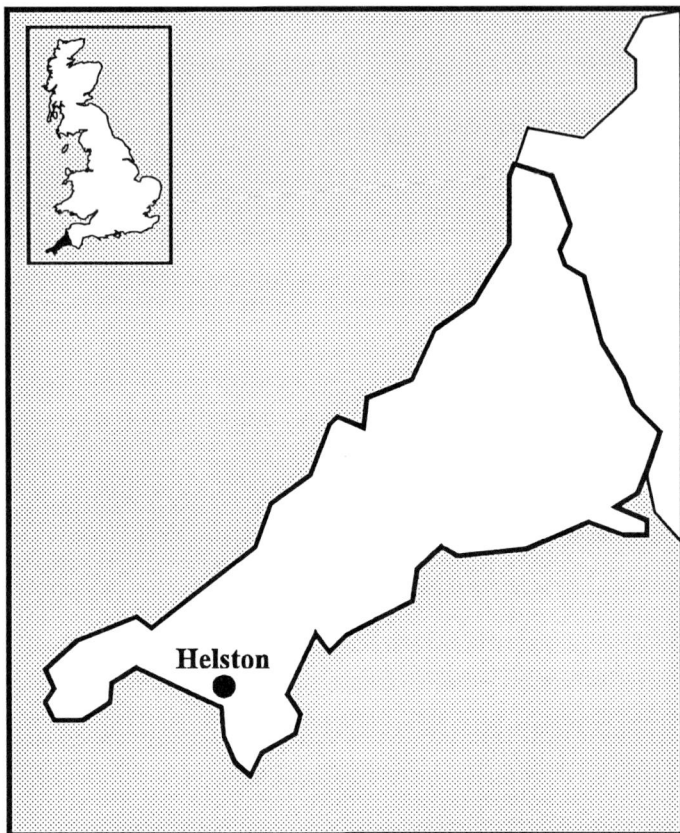

Helston

FLAMBARDS VICTORIAN VILLAGE

CULDROSE MANOR
HELSTON
CORNWALL TR13 OGA

TELEPHONE; 0326-574 549/573 404
OPEN: MONDAY - SUNDAY .... 10.00 - 5.00
        LAST ADMISSION FOR MUSEUM........................... 4.00
        PARK... 10.00 - 5.30.
        EARLY APRIL TO END OCTOBER
ADMISSION: CHARGE

SHOP. REFRESHMENTS. TOILETS.

  ♿ DISABLED ACCESS TO ALL AREAS.

Near the naval air station at Culdrose is the Aero park with a collection of military aircraft, with easy access to the flight decks, a display of the Battle of Britain and a fully re-constructed Victorian village. In the village, which has shops, streets and horse-drawn carriages, are two chemist's shops and a dental surgery. One shop is an authentic recreation of a Victorian pharmacy complete with drug runs, coloured jars and bottles, patent medicines and pill making equipment. The other, The Unique Chemist's Shop Time Capsule, is an apothecaries shop that was closed in 1909, then locked away and forgotten until discovered in 1987. It has been re-assembled exactly as found! The dental surgery has a chair, foot pedal drill and assorted teeth extracting forceps. The 'Britain in the Blitz' recreates a street during the Second World War.

In the Penwith Peninsular is the enigmatic monument, the Men-an-Tol stones. Although no longer in their original location, legend says that, if babies are passed through the hole in the stone, they will not suffer from rickets.

Cumbria

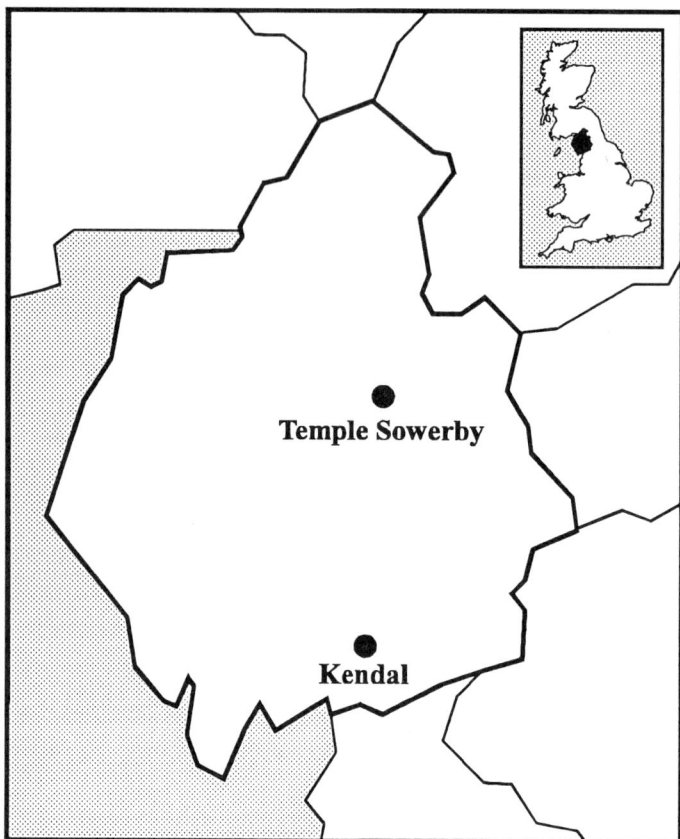

ABBOT HALL ART GALLERY & KENDAL MUSEUM OF LAKELAND LIFE & INDUSTRY

KENDAL
CUMBRIA LA9 5AL

TELEPHONE: 0539-722 464
OPEN: MONDAY - SATURDAY ....10.30 - 5.00
              SUNDAY ....2.00 - 5.00
ADMISSION: CHARGE
SHOP. TOILETS.

 ♿ DISABLED ACCESS TO ART GALLERY & GROUND FLOOR OF MUSEUM ONLY.

Abbot Hall was restored and converted into an art gallery in the late 1950's and houses a fine collection of period and contemporary works, including those of George Romney, John Ruskin, Ben Nicholson, John Piper and Elizabeth Frink. The stables now house the Museum of Lakeland Life and Industry and a recent 'street scene' includes a reconstructed late nineteenth century pharmacy with a drug run of bottles and jars, pill making equipment and prescription books. An unusual shop is the Marks and Spencer penny bazaar, fore-runner of to-day's multi-million pound chain, a draper's shop and photographic shop. Upstairs is a room devoted to Arthur Ransome and a delightful farm parlour and bedroom.

ACORN BANK GARDEN

TEMPLE SOWERBY
NR. PENRITH
CUMBRIA CA10 1SP

☏ TELEPHONE: 07683-61893
OPEN: MONDAY - SUNDAY ....10.00 -6.00
                1ST APRIL - 1ST NOVEMBER
ADMISSION TO THE HOUSE BY WRITTEN APPLICATION TO THE SUE RYDER FOUNDATION
ADMISSION: CHARGE, NATIONAL TRUST
SHOP. PLANTS FOR SALE. TOILETS. REFRESHMENTS.
♿ DISABLED ACCESS.

The red sandstone house is let to the Sue Ryder Foundation but the 2.5 acre garden is managed by the National Trust and is open from Spring to Autumn. Protected by fine oaks, under which grow a large display of daffodils, the garden has orchards, mixed borders planted with shrubs, roses and herbaceous plants and the most extensive collection of herbs in the north including American and English physic plants. These are closely planted in three long south-west facing beds and have many unusual varieties.

Derbyshire

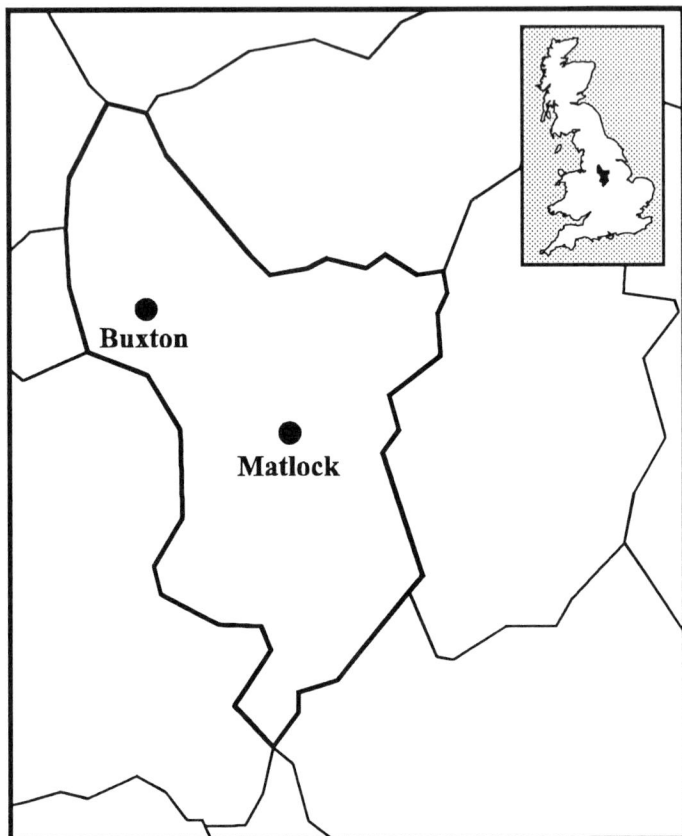

BUXTON MUSEUM & ART GALLERY

TERRACE ROAD
BUXTON
DERBYSHIRE SK17 6DJ

TELEPHONE: 0298-24658
OPEN: TUESDAY - FRIDAY...9.30 - 5.30
            SATURDAY..9.30 - 5.00
ADMISSION: CHARGE
SHOP. REFRESHMENTS. TOILETS.

DISABLED ACCESS TO ALL MUSEUM.

Nestling 1,000 feet above sea level in the Derbyshire Hills, Buxton owes its fame to the thermal springs which bubble up at a constant 28°C. It is still possible to sample the waters from St Ann's Well, opposite the Crescent, the town's most elegant building. The Pavilion, Gardens and Octagon concert hall, which date from the late 1800's, still form the nucleus of the town's leisure activities and include Serpentine walks through landscaped gardens, a swimming pool filled with the warm spa waters, and the winding river Wye.

The Museum, which has a large natural history display and a gallery called 'The Wonders of the Peaks' has also a collection of photographs depicting the Spa town in its hey-day. A book by John Leach on the History of Buxton can be purchased in the museum.

THE PAVILION

SOUTH PARADE
MATLOCK BATH
DERBYSHIRE DE4 3NR

℡ TELEPHONE: 0629 55082
    OPEN: MONDAY - SUNDAY ....9.30 - 5.30
              MARCH - OCTOBER
              OTHER..10.00 - 4.00
              CLOSED TUESDAY
              NOVEMBER - FEBRUARY
    ADMISSION: FREE
    SHOP.
♿ DISABLED ACCESS.

The town owes its name to the baths originally built to take advantage of the warm thermal springs which rise from the depths to emerge at a constant 20°C. The former hydropathic hotel on Matlock Bank, built in 1852, now accommodates the County Council. Although there is no museum chronicling the history of the spa town the calciferous waters can still be taken from one of the original well pumps in the Pavilion, which is now home to the Tourist Information Centre and Mining Museum.

The surrounding area is famous for the unique well dressing ceremonies - a thanksgiving for water - notable for its purity.

The Records Office in New Street has some interesting minutes, accounts and photographs of Smedley's Hydropathic Establishment 1859-1955, the Buxton Thermal Baths 1935-1956, the Rockside Hydro's plans and inventories 1900-1946, and the Tor House Hydro sale catalogue 1927. Open 9.30-1.00 & 2.00-4.45, telephone: 0629-580 000 ext. 7347.

Devon

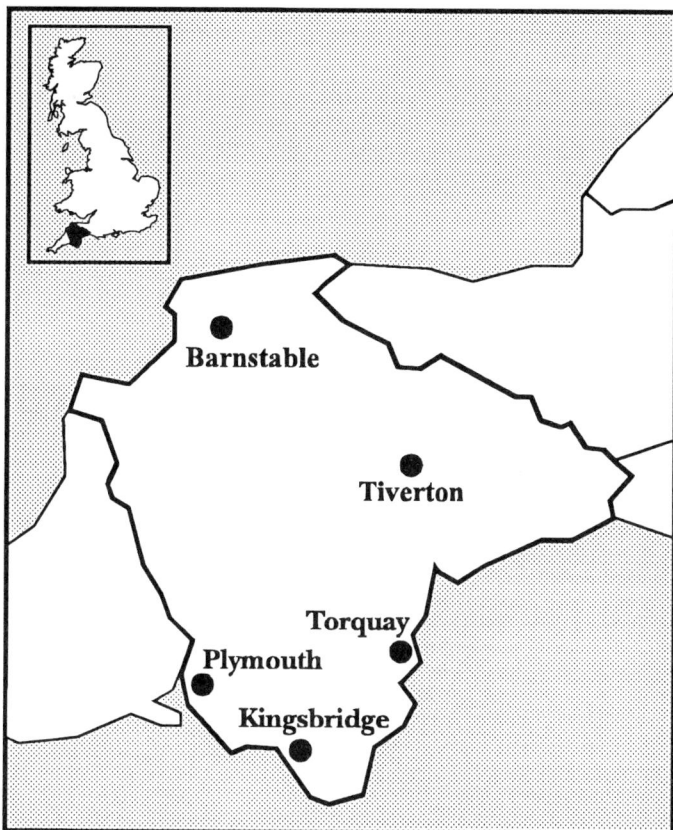

MUSEUM OF NORTH DEVON

THE SQUARE
BARNSTAPLE
DEVON EX32 8LN

☎ TELEPHONE: 0271-46747
OPEN: TUESDAY - SATURDAY ....10.00 - 4.30
ADMISSION: FREE
SHOP.

♿ DISABLED ACCESS.

The museum displays the natural history of North Devon together with displays on early man, archaeology and the trade and industry of the area with special relation to the local pottery making. The medical collections are derived mostly from the company of Arthur H. Cox & Co. Ltd. established in Brighton in 1839 but now based in Barnstaple. They include Dr. Mackenzie's anti-catarrhal smelling salts, 1900; a collection of Wedgwood and other stoneware pestles and mortars, 1890; prescription book of Joseph B. Harris 1875-1883; Dr. Forbes thermometer, 1900. Not on display but available by prior appointment is a priced catalogue of coated pills, 1890 and reproductions of Cox's showcard system, 1930.

COOKWORTHY MUSEUM

THE OLD GRAMMAR SCHOOL
108 FORE STREET
KINGSBRIDGE
DEVON

☎ TELEPHONE: 0548-853 235
    OPEN: MONDAY - SATURDAY .... 10.00 - 5.00
             LAST ENTRY 4.30
             EASTER - SEPTEMBER
             MONDAY - FRIDAY .... 10.30 - 4.00
             OCTOBER
    ADMISSION: CHARGE
    SHOP. CRAFT DEMONSTRATIONS.
& DISABLED ACCESS TO GROUND FLOOR & GARDEN. (RING FIRST).
† GROUPS ADVANCED BOOKING.

The museum is named after William Cookworthy who was born in Kingsbridge in 1705. A Quaker, and an apothecary, he discovered china clay in Cornwall and became the first Englishman to make true porcelain. William was probably a scholar at the 17th century Grammar School which has now become the museum and contains examples of the china he made and the story of china clay. The rural life of South Devon is well displayed in the farm gallery and dairy with everything from costumes to toys. There is also a large collection of photographs illustrating the life and times of the South Hams. A pharmacy, typical of the turn of the century, shows the drug runs, pill-making equipment, bottles, jars, pots of ointment and pills which according to the labels cured everything from headaches to varicose veins.

AMBULANCE MUSEUM

WATERLOO CLOSE
STONEHOUSE
PLYMOUTH
DEVON PL1 3ST

℡ TELEPHONE: 0752-266 851
OPEN: MONDAY - SATURDAY....................................9.00 - 5.00
ADMISSION: CHARGE
SHOP. TOILETS.

♿ DISABLED ACCESS TO ALL THE MUSEUM.

This unique museum, all under cover, contains 55 ambulances dating from 1830 to 1989, memorabilia from 1814 to 1990 and film archives from 1899 to 1990. There are also photographs and records from 600A.D. to 1990.

TIVERTON MUSEUM

ST. ANDREW STREET
TIVERTON
DEVON EX16 6PH

℡ TELEPHONE: 0884-256 295
OPEN: MONDAY - SATURDAY.................................10.30 - 4.30
ADMISSION: FREE
SHOP.

The museum aims to display the life and history of the town and adjacent environs from pre-history to modern times. The agricultural hall has a wide range of farm implements while the Alfold Gallery has farm wagons and horse drawn vehicles including a reconstructed smithy. The Authers Gallery has the 'Tivvy Bumper', a G.W.R. tank engine, which was used on the branch line. A lace machine, which was still in use until 1975, is there to show the local industry and examples of lace which has been used by Royal brides since Queen Victoria.

The medical items include a tooth key, leech jar, Victorian hearing aid, voice conducting ear cornet, ear syringe, eye dropper and nasal douche; 19th century medicine chest with labelled bottles, Maw's improved domestic machine for constipation of 1840; craniotomy forceps from 1871; various medicine bottles, jars and pill making equipment; a doctor's bag and dentist's chair, foot drill, spittoon, lamp, articulator and instruments.

BYGONES

FORE STREET
ST. MARYCHURCH
TORQUAY
DEVON TQ1 4PR

☎ TELEPHONE: 0803-326 108
 OPEN: MONDAY - SUNDAY .... 10.00 - 5.00
                EXTENDED OPENING .... 10.00 - 10.00
                JUNE - SEPTEMBER
                LAST ENTRY ONE HOUR BEFORE CLOSING
        ADMISSION: CHARGE
        SHOP. REFRESHMENTS. TOILETS.
♿ DISABLED ACCESS TO THE STREET.

Housed in a disused cinema, the owners Mr. and Mrs. Cuming have brought together a fascinating collection of memorabilia and artefacts displayed in a charming Victorian street of shops and work rooms. The Apothecary's shop has items from a local chemist, Mr. Franks, dating from about 1880, together with pill making equipment, bottles of assorted colours, some containing the original potions and perfumes and various proprietary medicines. A dentist's surgery has the chair and foot treadle drill and cupboard for the instruments. The railway museum has life size and model exhibits.

TORQUAY MUSEUM

529 BABBACOMBE ROAD
TORQUAY
DEVON TQ1 1HG

ⓓ TELEPHONE: 0803-293 975
OPEN: MONDAY - SATURDAY..................................10.00 - 4.45
SUNDAYS ONLY ....2.00 - 2.45
JULY-MID SEPTEMBER
LIMITED OPENING IN WINTER
ADMISSION: CHARGE
SHOP. TOILETS. SCHOOLROOM FOR HANDLING OBJECTS.
TALKS & SLIDES.

ⓓ DISABLED ACCESS RESTRICTED.(STAIRCASE).

🏃 GROUP BOOKINGS ON SATURDAY BY ARRANGEMENT.

Owned by the Torquay Natural History Society and opened in 1876 the museum is divided between 6 exciting galleries. The archaeological gallery shows the development of man and includes the oldest human remains yet to be discovered in Britain. From fossils to Victoriana the museum explains the local history with a wide range of artefacts. In 1891 one of the world's most famous writer's of detective fiction, Agatha Christie, was born in Torquay and a fascinating display of memorabilia commemorates her centenary. Pharmaceutical bygones are shown in an upper gallery including a glass percolator used for making tinctures, a plaster iron, a rice paper cachet machine, morstacht cachets, two leech holders, a silver spatula, a pill making machine and assorted glass bottles and jars.

Dorset

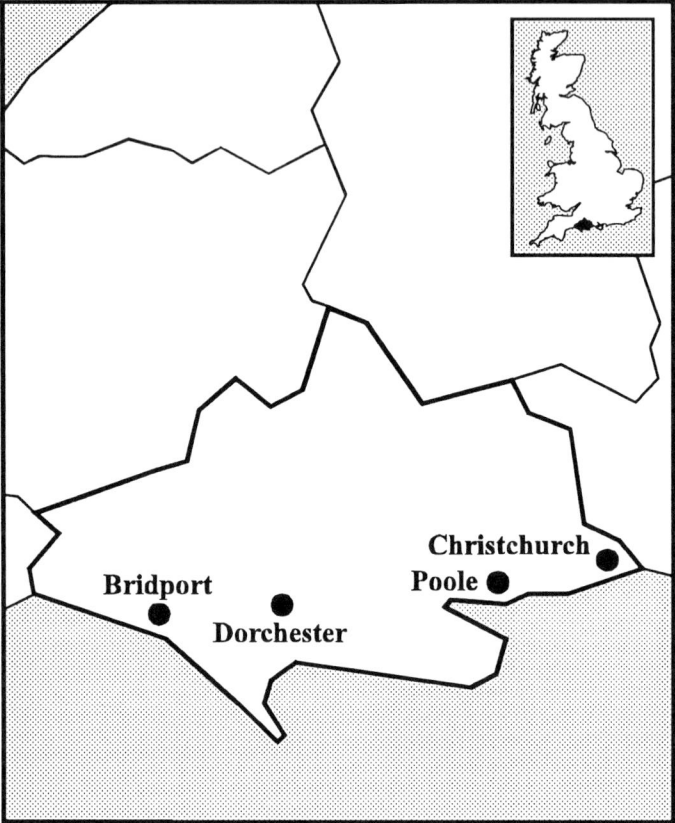

BRIDPORT MUSEUM

SOUTH STREET
BRIDPORT
DORSET

TELEPHONE: 0308-22116
OPEN: MONDAY - SATURDAY ....10.00 - 4.30
             SUNDAY ....2.00 - 4.30
             SATURDAY SUNDAY ONLY
             NOVEMBER - EASTER WEDNESDAY
ADMISSION: CHARGE
SHOP.

   ♿   DISABLED ACCESS GROUND FLOOR ONLY.

   🏃   SCHOOL PARTIES BY APPOINTMENT ANY TIME.

This delightful local history museum is housed in a fine Tudor building and tells the story of the rope and net making industry which made the town so famous. The medical items on display include a dozen drug jars and Victorian weighing scales and bottles, Woodville's Medical Botany book and an oil painting of Dr. Giles Robert's, known locally as the 'poor man's friend'. He lived from 1780 - 1840 and was involved in a movement to provide care for the poor. There is a box file of reference notes on him and his work which is available from the curator.

RED HOUSE MUSEUM, ART GALLERY & GARDENS

       QUAY ROAD
       CHRISTCHURCH
       DORSET BH23 1BU

  📞   TELEPHONE: 0202-482 860
       OPEN: MONDAY - SATURDAY.....................................1.00 - 5.00
                SUNDAY...2.00 - 5.00
       ADMISSION: CHARGE
       SHOP. TOILETS.

   ♿   DISABLED ACCESS TO GROUND FLOOR AND GARDEN.

   🏃   GROUPS BY ARRANGEMENT.

An elegant Georgian house just a few minutes from the River Stour provides a fascinating glimpse into the past life of Christchurch. Reconstructed scenes in the new archaeology galleries, domestic bygones, dolls, toys and artefacts from local industries, such as the small detailed fusee watch chain making, marine and fishing, natural history dioramas, costumes and an Art Gallery of temporary exhibitions make this well displayed museum an exciting place to visit.

The walled garden provides a quiet, peaceful oasis with herbaceous borders, old roses, woodland walk and formal herb and physic garden. The plants in the physic garden

include angelica, apothecary's rose, bay, betony, elecampane, evening primrose, feverfew, fleabane, good King Henry,
hop, lemon balm, lungwort, monkshood, mugwort, periwinkle, rue, sage, selfheal, St. John's wort and thyme. A
leaflet of the plants with their uses and a short description
each should be available in 1993.

DORSET COUNTY MUSEUM

HIGH WEST STREET
DORCHESTER
DORSET

☎ TELEPHONE: 0305-262 735
OPEN: MONDAY - SATURDAY .... 10.00 - 5.00
ADMISSION: CHARGE
SHOP.

♿ DISABLED ACCESS TO GROUND FLOOR ONLY.

Founded in 1846 and run by the Dorset Natural History
and Archaeological Society the museum is concerned with
anything under, on or above ground in the county of Dorset
in the past, present or future. Housed in a magnificent iron
Victorian gallery the geology, natural history and archaeology sections show the wealth of early history uncovered in
the area. Thomas Hardy's study is reconstructed as it was
when he lived and worked at Max Gate and has the largest
collection of his manuscripts, books from his own library and
many of his personal possessions. In the Victorian Gallery is
a surgeon's cabinet, used at Bridport Hospital, containing
cupping equipment, 17th and 18th century medicine bottles
and 19th century pharmacists' jars. In the reserve collection
(by appointment only) are further pharmacists' pill making
equipment, a medicine book, tools and bottles, post-mortem
hammer, rheumatism relief machine and a 19th century
dentist's drill.

The museum has also some interesting leaflets on
medical men connected with the town. Thomas Sydenham
1624-1689, the 'English Hippocrates and master of clinical
medicine'; Benjamin Jesty, 1737-1816, the pre-Jennerian
vaccinator; Sir Frederick Treves, 1853-1923, who achieved

fame as a notable surgeon and writer, and H.G.J. Moseley who helped Rutherford in the discovery of atomic numbers.

WATERFRONT MUSEUM

POOLE QUAY
POOLE
DORSET BH15 1BW

☎ TELEPHONE: 0202-675151 EXT. 202
OPEN: MONDAY - SATURDAY................................10.00 - 5.00
            SUNDAY...2.00 - 5.00
CLOSED: CHRISTMAS DAY, BOXING DAY, NEW YEAR'S DAY,
            GOOD FRIDAY
ADMISSION: CHARGE
TOILETS. SHOP.

  ♿ DISABLED ACCESS EXCEPT TO TOWN CELLARS.

Waterfront brings Poole's colourful seafaring past to life in two historic buildings. The Victorian street scene has the Old Curiosity Shop, White Hart Pub and Cartledge's Pharmacy. Most of the fixtures and fittings date from the shop's establishment in 1879, including the counter, display cases, shelf units and pediments and labelled drawer units. The shelves are stocked with runs of contemporary and later drug jars and containers. The dispensing equipment includes pill-makers, measures, scales and pestles and mortars. The top floor traces the history of Scouting from its small beginning on nearby Brownsea Island to a world-wide organisation.

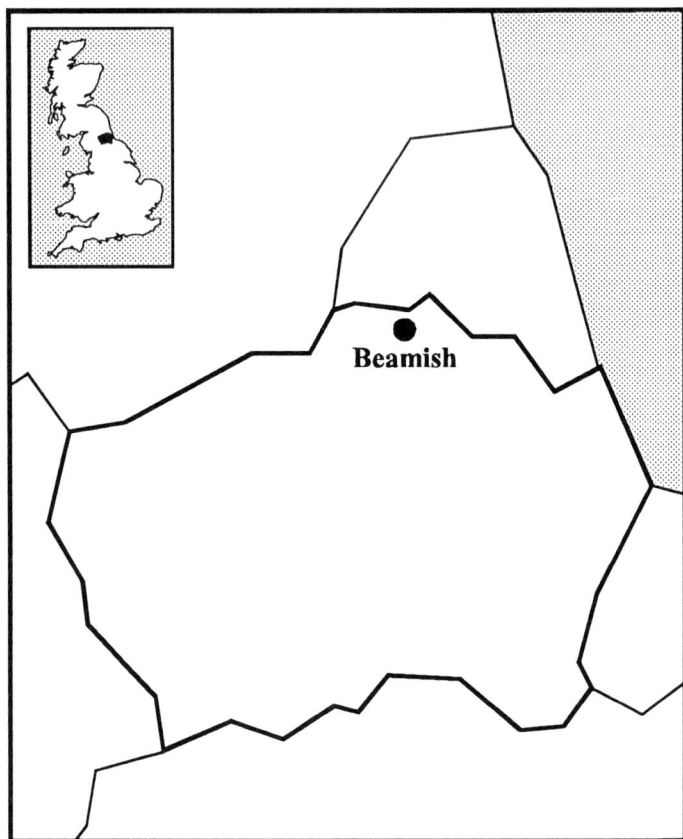

BEAMISH, THE NORTH OF ENGLAND OPEN AIR MUSEUM

BEAMISH HALL
STANLEY
DURHAM DH9 ORG

☽ TELEPHONE: 0207-231 811
OPEN: MONDAY - SUNDAY ....10.00 - 6.00
LATE MARCH TO END OCTOBER
TUESDAY - SUNDAY...................................10.00 - 5.00
IN WINTER MONTHS
PERIOD AREAS CLOSE...5.45

LAST GUIDED TOUR OF DRIFT MINE 5.30
ADMISSION: CHARGE
SHOP. REFRESHMENTS. TOILETS.

☾ DISABLED ACCESS TO MANY AREAS.

🕺 PARTY GROUP VISITS AND EDUCATIONAL VISITS TO PRE-BOOK.

Created in 1970 and covering 200 acres of woodland and rolling countryside the Beamish is preserving the heritage of the North East by rescuing buildings from all over the region and rebuilding them as a living town and work place. All the buildings are fitted out with appropriate objects and machinery. Costumed staff skilfully explain their function and the way people lived in the town in the years immediately before the First World War. The museum is divided into areas joined by footpaths; the town, the railway station, the transport collection, the home farm, the pit cottages and the colliery. In the town the dentist practices from his own home. The waiting room resembles his front parlour, the surgery is upstairs with the cast iron chair, foot treadle drill and cylinders of nitrous oxide. In the technician's workshop sets of false teeth are being made. Further exhibits are in store such as a doctor's surgery and many instruments from the 1920's and 1930's. The reference library has a number of old textbooks on medicine and medical history, a good collection of medical supplies and dentistry trade catalogues and a large photographic library.

Essex

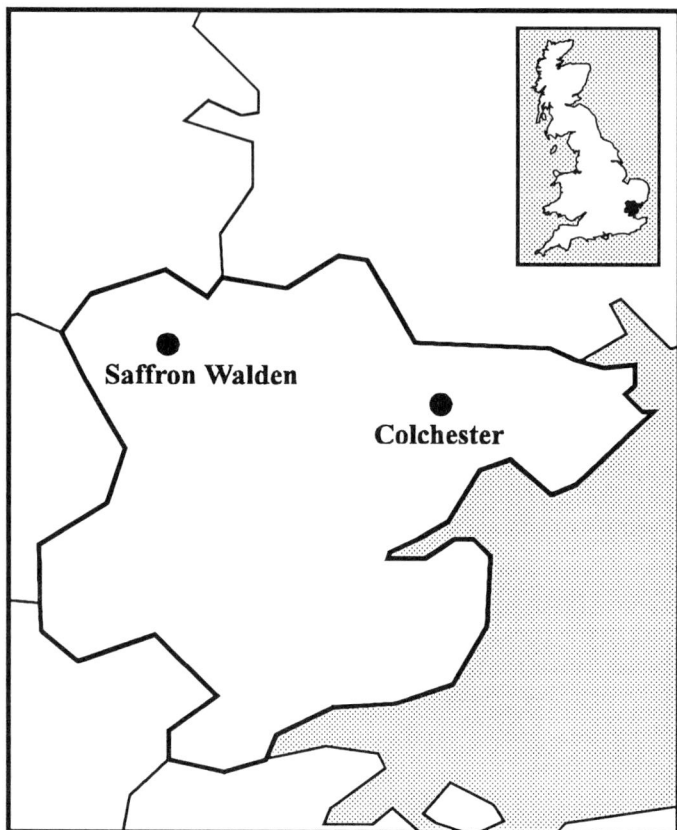

COLCHESTER MUSEUM

THE CASTLE
COLCHESTER
ESSEX CO1 1TJ

☾ TELEPHONE: 0206-712 222
    OPEN: MONDAY - SATURDAY .... 10.00 - 5.00
               SUNDAY .... 2.00 - 5.00
               APRIL - SEPTEMBER
               MONDAY - FRIDAY .... 10.00 - 5.00
               SATURDAY.. 10.00 - 4.00
               OCTOBER - MARCH
    ADMISSION: CHARGE

SHOP. TOILETS.

  ♿ DISABLED ACCESS TO WHOLE MUSEUM.

The castle at Colchester is one of the oldest in the country, built in 1076 on the foundations of an earlier Roman temple. The museum is in the keep and has new Roman galleries displaying archaeological material from sites in Essex. Amongst these are some medical items such as spoon probes and instrument handles. Later medical items of the 19th century including ear-trumpets, travelling medicine chests, bottles and other pharmacy equipment are not on display, so please ring to make an appointment first.

SAFFRON WALDEN MUSEUM

MUSEUM STREET
SAFFRON WALDEN
ESSEX CB10 1JL

  ☎ TELEPHONE: 0799-522 494
       OPEN: MONDAY - SATURDAY.................................10.00 - 5.00
                 SUNDAY..2.30 - 5.00
                 APRIL TO END OCTOBER
                 TUESDAY - SATURDAY ....11.00 - 4.00
                 SUNDAY..2.30 - 4.30
                 NOVEMBER TO END MARCH
       ADMISSION: CHARGE
       SHOP. REFRESHMENTS. TOILETS.

  ♿ DISABLED ACCESS TO WHOLE MUSEUM.

This Victorian building has interesting displays of archaeology, ceramics, glass and local history. A costume gallery shows the clothes and accessories of the 18th and 19th centuries. The Egyptian gallery has mummies of a small boy, a cat and canopic jars for the internal organs. There are 2 skeletons from a Saxon cemetery which were exhumed in 1875, one has an axe cut on the back of the skull which was possibly surgical. There are some Dutch drug jars on display but other medical items including various electrical appliances, nasal irrigators, medical cabinets and some contents of a chemist's shop are in the reserve collection available on application to the keeper of Social History.

Gloucestershire

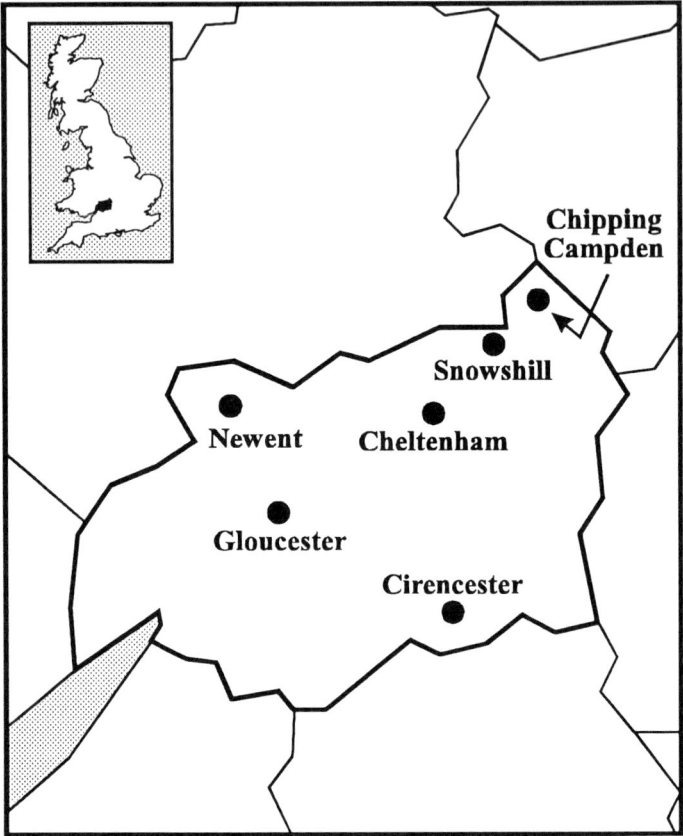

THE JENNER MUSEUM

THE CHANTRY
CHURCH LANE
BERKELEY
GLOUCESTERSHIRE GL13 9BH

TELEPHONE: 0453-810 631
OPEN: TUESDAY - SATURDAY & B.H. MONDAY
                APRIL - SEPTEMBER .... 12.30 - 5.30
                SUNDAY .... 1.00 - 5.30
ADMISSION: CHARGE
SHOP.

Edward Jenner was born in Berkeley on 17 May 1749, a son of the then vicar. He was a student at St George's Hospital, London and a pupil of the great surgeon, John Hunter. He settled as a country doctor in Berkeley, joined local medical societies, contributed papers on heart disease, and recorded one of the earliest accounts of hypothermia. Jenner's interest in the link between cowpox and smallpox had begun during the years of his apprenticeship to Dr. Daniel Ludlow at Chipping Sodbury, and eventually resulted in his discovery of vaccination against smallpox. He died at the Chantry and is buried in the church next door. In the grounds of the house he had a rustic thatched hut which he called the Temple of Vaccinia, where he vaccinated the poor free of charge. The museum contains Jenner's personal possessions and work and some relics from James Phipps, the boy he first vaccinated. A conference centre, converted from the adjoining Coach House, was funded by Mr. Ryoichi Sasakawa, a Japanese philanthropist, and offers an ideal location for conferences and meetings of all descriptions.

PITTVILLE PUMP ROOM & GALLERY OF FASHION

PITTVILLE PARK
CHELTENHAM
GLOUCESTERSHIRE

☎ TELEPHONE: 0242-512 740
OPEN: TUESDAY - SUNDAY ....10.30 - 5.00
APRIL - OCTOBER
TUESDAY - SATURDAY ....10.30 - 5.00
NOVEMBER - MARCH
ADMISSION: CHARGE
TOILETS.

&. DISABLED ACCESS TO GROUND FLOOR.

⚐ GUIDED TOURS BY PRIOR ARRANGEMENT.

Lying in the heart of the Cotswolds, Cheltenham's saline spring was discovered over 250 years ago. In 1738, Captain Skillicome deepened the well, erected a cover and then built an adjacent ballroom and billiard room to encourage visitors. During the next 100 years scores more medicinal springs were discovered and other pump-rooms built, including the magnificent Pittville, set in a lovely park. After a chequered history and creeping decay the Pump Room was restored in 1960 to its former glory and is in use most evenings for private and public functions. Spa water is still available, being pumped to the fountain in the main hall from a well 80ft deep. The 'waters' can also be taken in the Town Hall.

The Gallery of Fashion is a visual presentation of the town from the late 18th century to the Swinging Sixties with a fascinating collection of jewellery showing the changing taste from Regency to Art Nouveau including a spectacular collection of tiaras.

WOOLSTAPLERS HALL MUSEUM

HIGH STREET
CHIPPING CAMPDEN
GLOUCESTERSHIRE GL55 6HB

ⓓ TELEPHONE: 0386-840 289
OPEN: MONDAY - SUNDAY .... 11.00 - 6.00
            1ST APRIL - 31ST OCTOBER
ADMISSION: CHARGE
SHOP.

 &. NO DISABLED ACCESS.

The Hall is thought to have been built in 1340 by a local family where the wool merchants did their buying and selling. Today it has a varied collection of domestic bygones, typewriters, early cameras, man-traps, a 19th century wood-worker's tools, the contents of a local cobbler's shop, some equipment from a 1920's cinema and an apothecary's shop. The contents come from many different sources and include the coloured glass bottles, jars, ointment pots, pill making equipment and drug run from the turn of the century.

CORINIUM MUSEUM

PARK STREET
CIRENCESTER
GLOUCESTERSHIRE GL7 2BX

☎ TELEPHONE: 0285-655 611
    OPEN: MONDAY - SATURDAY.................................10.00 - 5.30
                SUNDAY...2.00 - 5.30
    ADMISSION: CHARGE
    SHOP. TOILETS.
♿ DISABLED ACCESS TO WHOLE MUSEUM.

The Roman town of Corinium became the second largest town in Britain and the museum contains many important objects from that time. These include a fully reconstructed Roman kitchen, triclinium (dining room) and the workshop of a stonemason or mosaic craftsman. The 'hare' and 'hunting dogs' mosaics are in the museum with tombstones, a Corinthian capital, 'the Septimus Stone' and some Romano-British medical instruments. These finds are extremely rare and the museum is fortunate to have 2 bronze scalpel handles with the remains of their iron blades, a number of bronze spatula/probes which are probably medical and 2 bronze retractors.

Other displays include Saxon and Medieval galleries, the Cotswold wool trade and the history of Cirencester from Tudor to modern times.

FOLK MUSEUM

99 - 103 WESTGATE STREET
GLOUCESTER
GLOUCESTERSHIRE

☎ TELEPHONE: 0452-526 467
    OPEN: MONDAY - SATURDAY.................................10.00 - 5.00
                SUNDAY...10.00 - 4.00
                JULY - SEPTEMBER ONLY
    ADMISSION: FREE
    SHOP. TOILETS. EXHIBITIONS.
♿ DISABLED ACCESS TO GROUND FLOOR AND COURTYARD.

Three timber-framed houses are the home of the Folk Museum which displays the local industries, crafts and work of the people of Gloucester. A double Gloucester dairy, ironmonger, wheelwright, cobbler and carpenter's workshops, exhibits of the horn industry and brass pin making, domestic bygones, glass and ceramics are on display.

In the reserve collection are surgeon's and general practitioner's books which can be seen on application to the curator.

MUSEUM OF ADVERTISING & PACKAGING

THE ALBERT WAREHOUSE
GLOUCESTER DOCKS
GLOUCESTER GL1 2EH

☎ TELEPHONE: 0452-302 309
OPEN: TUESDAY - SUNDAY .... 10.00 - 6.00
CLOSED: DURING WEEKDAYS IN WINTER 5.00
ADMISSION: CHARGE
EVENING BOOKINGS BY SPECIAL ARRANGEMENT.
SHOP. REFRESHMENTS. TOILETS.

&. DISABLED ACCESS.

ᕏ GROUPS BY ARRANGEMENT.

Robert Opie started his collection of advertising and packaging over 25 years ago and today it is the first museum of its kind with over 300,000 items relating to the history of our consumer society. The packets, tins, bottles, posters and display cards show a vast range of goods from cigarettes, shoe polish, cereals, soap powders, spirits and biscuits to patent medicines from 1880 - 1990.

At the rear of the museum is a chemist's shop with mahogany drug run, cash till, dispensing area with mirror and some medical items. The patent medicines and related health items show the popularity of 'cure all' remedies.

The imaginative changing displays show a grocer's shop filled with goods available for one particular year, an individual brand showing its development through a decade and a WW2 shop with the toys, games, comics, posters and ration books of that period.

The museum is hoping to increase its exhibition space in the mid 1990's.

THE SHAMBLES

CHURCH STREET
NEWENT
GLOUCESTERSHIRE

☎ TELEPHONE: 0531-822 144
OPEN: TUESDAY - SUNDAY ....10.00 - 6.00
MARCH - OCTOBER (DUSK IF EARLIER)
CLOSED: MONDAY (EXCEPT BANK HOLIDAY)
ADMISSION: CHARGE
TOILETS. REFRESHMENTS. SHOP.

 ♿ DISABLED ACCESS.

Hidden behind the bustling streets of this country town lies a staggeringly large collection of over thirty trade shops set round cobbled streets, alleys and squares, a complete town capturing the atmosphere of Victorian life. The Doctor's Dispensary and Chemist's shop of the 1920's displays drug jars, apothecary's scales, pill making machines, skeletons, amputation sets, and electric shock machines.

SNOWSHILL MANOR

NR. BROADWAY
GLOUCESTERSHIRE WR12 7JU

☎ TELEPHONE: 0386-852 410
OPEN: WEDNESDAY - SUNDAY & B.H. MONDAY
....11.00 - 1.00 & 2.00 - 6.00
MAY - END SEPTEMBER
SATURDAY & SUNDAY ....11.00 - 1.00 & 2.00 - 5.00
APRIL & OCTOBER & EASTER SAT., SUN. & MON.
LAST ADMISSION 1/2 HOUR. BEFORE CLOSING
ADMISSION: CHARGE, NATIONAL TRUST
SHOP. TOILETS.

🚶 SCHOOL PARTIES BY APPOINTMENT.

The Manor was owned by Winchcombe Abbey until 1539 when it passed to the Crown. Since then it has had a number of owners and tenants until 1919, when in a semi-derelict state it was bought and restored by Charles Paget Wade. Wade was an architect, artist and craftsman from Yoxford in Suffolk, who inherited sugar estates in the West Indies from his father. This enabled him to devote his life to amassing his enormous and varied collection of craftsmanship from 1900 -1951, when he bequeathed what is a study collection to the National Trust.

The house is filled with an amazing collection of exhibits from Japanese Samurai warriors, bone-shaker bicycles, toys, and spinning wheels to Javanese dancing masks, musical instruments, and nautical and scientific objects. It involves a treasure hunt to find the medical items but there is a pewter castor oil spoon, pill rolling machines, mahogany medicine chests complete with glass bottles, a medicine chest from the East Indies in the shape of a metal scorpion and wooden Beadle's staves from the Bridewell and Bethlem hospitals, St. Thomas's and St. Bartholomew's. Further cupping sets, fleams, scarifiers and medicine chests are available in the reserve collection, by appointment.

The beautiful gardens with walls, steps and alleys are terraced to provide enticing views and walkways.

Greater Manchester

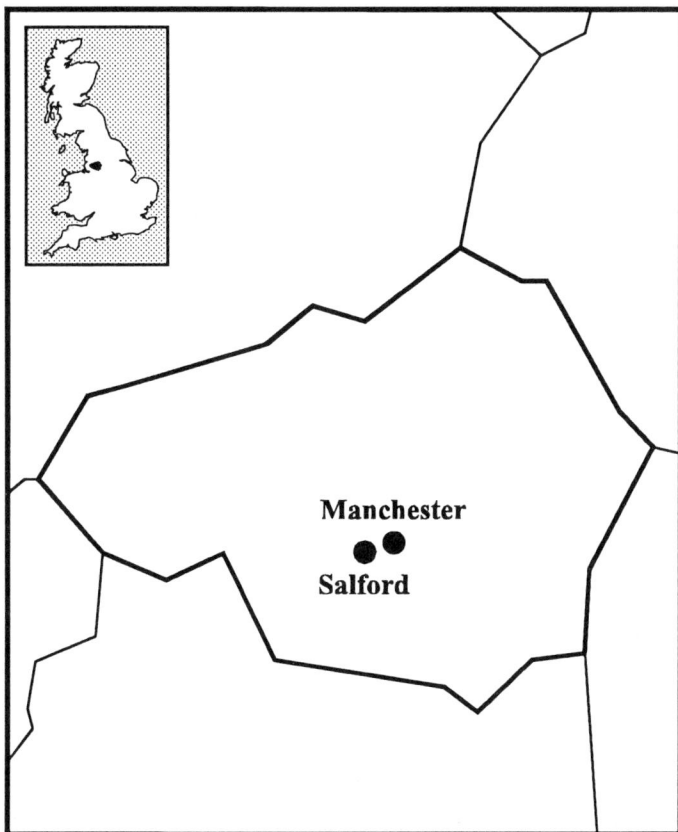

MUSEUM OF SCIENCE & INDUSTRY

LIVERPOOL ROAD
CASTLEFIELD
MANCHESTER
GREATER MANCHESTER M3 4JP

☏ TELEPHONE: 061-832 2244
OPEN: MONDAY - SUNDAY ....10.00 - 5.00
ADMISSION: CHARGE
SHOP. REFRESHMENTS. TOILETS.

♿ DISABLED ACCESS TO MOST PARTS OF MUSEUM.

ホホ GROUPS TO PRE BOOK 061-833 0027. CONFERENCE CENTRE 061-832 2244.

Located in 5 historic buildings on the site of the oldest passenger railway station in the world, the museum has 13 galleries covering everything from steam to space, transport to textiles. 'Microscopes in Manchester' features microscopes which were used for a variety of purposes, including medical ones. Some stored in the reserve collection were used at the Manchester Royal Infirmary and the Royal Eye Hospital between 1900 and 1960, such as an early Zeiss of 1899 and 1907, a compound 'Army' microscope by J. Swift & Son of 1917, and 4 'Bactil' microscopes from 1935 to 1963. 'Underground Manchester' deals with the broad theme of public health in relation to water supply, sewerage and sanitation systems. A reconstruction of a man-entry sewer using materials reclaimed from the 1830's Bridgewater Street sewer is complete with sounds and smells!

CITY OF SALFORD MUSEUM & ART GALLERY

PEEL PARK
SALFORD
GREATER MANCHESTER M5 4WU

☎ TELEPHONE: 061-736 2649
OPEN: MONDAY - FRIDAY .... 10.00 - 4.45
                 SUNDAY .... 2.00 - 5.00
ADMISSION: FREE
SHOP. TOILETS. REFRESHMENTS.

♿ DISABLED ACCESS TO ALL FLOORS.

An elegant Georgian mansion, Lark Hill, was built by James Ackers, the 'father of the silk trade' in the early 1790's. Found to be unsafe in 1935 it was demolished and a new wing opened in 1938. This now houses a display of fine and decorative arts including an outstanding collection of works by L.S. Lowry and frequent changing exhibitions. In 1955 the City Council decided to salvage features from the houses and shops being demolished in Salford and to recreate a small street within the museum. The street is named

'Lark Hill Place' after the original mansion and contains a tobacconist, pub, jeweller and pawnbroker, blacksmith, dressmaker, general store, music shop, printer's shop and period rooms. The chemist and druggist, John Hamer, was established in 1865 just six years before the first Act of Parliament regulating the buying, dispensing and selling of drugs and medicines was passed. Around the shop are a variety of drawers and storage jars, mortar and pestle, apothecaries' scales, a tongue scraper and Mather's balsamic plasters as used in the Scutari Hospital. Mrs. Driver, bleeder with leeches, had practised her trade until 1912. She obtained the leeches from a herb shop in Manchester and used them to treat black eyes and bruises.

Hampshire

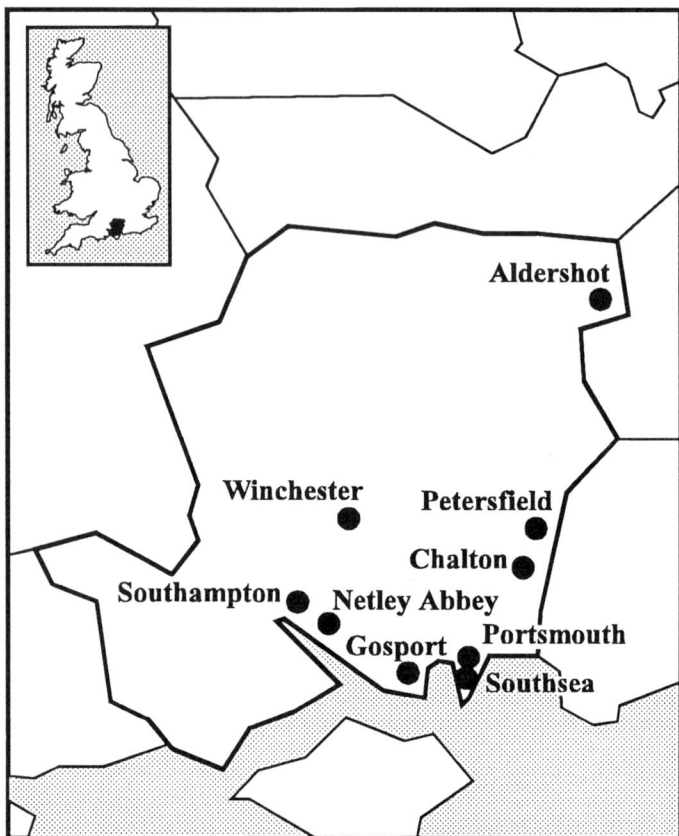

QUEEN ALEXANDRA'S ROYAL ARMY NURSING CORPS MUSEUM

ROYAL PAVILION
FARNBOROUGH ROAD
ALDERSHOT
HAMPSHIRE GU11 1PZ

TELEPHONE: 0252-349 315 (CURATOR)
                        0252-349 301 (MUSEUM)
OPEN: BY APPOINTMENT. WEEK DAYS ONLY.
ADMSSION: CHARGE
SHOP. CATERING BY ARRANGEMENT.

  ♿ DISABLED ACCESS BY ARRANGEMENT.

The museum was established in 1956 at Hindhead in Surrey and moved to the new training centre of the QARANC in 1967. At present its future is uncertain with the restructuring of the Army and reorganising of its property.

It was not until after the Crimean War and the work of Florence Nightingale and her band of nurses that the Queen authorised the appointment of trained civilian nurses in military hospitals. Between 1879 and 1902 the nurses served in the Zulu campaign, in North Africa and the Boer War.

In 1902, under the patronage of Queen Alexandra the service was augmented and redesigned calling itself Queen Alexandra's Imperial Military Nursing Service. During the first World War 10,000 trained nurses were serving and employed in casualty clearing stations in advance base hospitals. But it was the second World War that finally brought the nursing service into its own. In 1949 the nursing service finally became a regular corps of the British Army.

This excellent museum shows the history of the corps, from Florence Nightingale's carriage, which she used in the Crimea, to the Falklands, with models, photographs, equipment, letters, medals, uniforms, friendship cloths, the Canadian quilt and a cape worn by Sister McCallum with badges and flashes of patients, sewn into the lining during the Second World War

Archive material is available for research by appointment with the Curator.

ROYAL ARMY DENTAL CORPS MUSEUM

       HQ & CENTRAL GROUP RADC
       EVELYN WOODS ROAD
       ALDERSHOT
       HAMPSHIRE

  ☎ TELEPHONE: 0252-24431 EXT. 2782
      OPEN: MONDAY - FRIDAY .... 10.00 - 12.00 & 2.00 - 4.00
      ADMISSION: FREE
      SHOP.
  ♿ DISABLED ACCESS BY LIFT.

It was not until 1860 that dentists were recognised as a separate profession and in 1878 the first Dental Act was passed in Parliament, with the founding of the British Dental Association in 1880.

However since 1660 the soldier's teeth had been a constant source of problems for the Army. The regimental surgeons were required to preserve the soldier's teeth so that he could bite through the paper cartridge when loading his musket. Instruments to scale the teeth were issued for that purpose.

During the Boer War the British troops received dental attention in the field for the first time and some reminders of the frailty of vulcanite dentures when confronted with a trek ox and army biscuit diet are on display. There is a case covering World War 1 with drawings by Tonks of facial injuries. The high proportion of head wounds that resulted from trench warfare exposed the value of the dentist's services and led to the formation of the Army Dental Corps in 1921. The development of facio-maxillary surgery from these wounds is well displayed with the work of such men as Harold Gillies and William Kelsy.

The exploits of individuals, either captured and sent to Colditz or escaping from Poland, together with details of campaigns in North Africa, the Middle East and Europe are on display. From the Far East to Kenya and the Falklands, (an Argentinian dental chair is on display) the dental service has been active and especially more recently in the Gulf War.

ROYAL ARMY MEDICAL CORPS HISTORICAL MUSEUM

KEOGH BARRACKS
ASH VALE
ALDERSHOT
HAMPSHIRE GU12 5RQ

℡ TELEPHONE: 0252-24431 EXT. 5212
OPEN: MONDAY - FRIDAY .... 8.30 - 4.00
          WEEKENDS BY APPOINTMENT ONLY
ADMISSION: FREE

SHOP. TOILETS.

  ♿ DISABLED ACCESS.

The museum traces its origin back to the Army Medical School at Fort Pitt Chatham in the mid 19th century, later to Netley and finally to the College at Millbank. The contents were dispersed in World War 2, with some items lost by enemy action. It was reformed in 1951 at the RAMC depot.

The Medical Service itself is unique, having taken part in every campaign and battle which the British Army has waged since 1660, although the the Medical Corps was not formed until 23rd June 1898. The museum is arranged chronologically with the first exhibits from 1660-1854. They include early surgeons instruments, drawings by Sir Charles Bell from the battle of Waterloo, the Duke of Wellington's hearing aids, Napoleon's dental instruments and the story of Dr. James Barry - was he a woman?

The next section from 1854-57 deals with the Crimean War; the section from 1858-97 explains the formation of the Red Cross and shows bullet extractors, post-mortem instruments and a quilt made by Queen Victoria.

The Martin-Leake Medal room has citations and action prints of the 31 VC's awarded to the Army Medical Services. The Boer War and World War 1 has instruments, pills and medicines, stretcher bearers, gas masks and medical and surgical panniers and a section from 1920-45 has amongst its collection part of the original growth of penicillin cultured by Alexander Fleming who was in the RAMC in the First World War. From 1946 the items come from Cyprus, Kenya, Borneo and the Falklands war.

The outside display has an armoured car and Austin K2 Ambulance; a newly appointed Chapel, much of whose interior has come from Netley, has a small Physic Garden along one wall.

The Muiniment Room housing records and documents is available to view by Historians on application to the curator.

BUSTER ARCHAEOLOGICAL FARM

BASCOMB COPSE
CHALTON LANE
NR. CHALTON
HAMPSHIRE

☎ TELEPHONE: 0705-598 838
OPEN: MONDAY - FRIDAY .... 10.00 - 5.00
SATURDAY .... 2.00 - 5.00
SUNDAY .... 10.00 - 5.00
APRIL TO END OCTOBER
MONDAY - FRIDAY .... 10.00 - 4.00
IST NOVEMBER - 3RD MARCH
ADMISSION: CHARGE
SHOP. PICNIC FACILITIES.

🚶 SCHOOL PARTIES AND GROUPS BY APPOINTMENT.

In 1968 a group of eminent archaeologists and others decided it would be interesting and useful to have a 'hands on facility' for children and adults to see the archaeological research into the agricultural economy of the Iron Age. In 1990 the farm moved to its present site and here you can see the buildings, charcoal clamps, iron smelting sheds, grain storage pits, crops and ancient breeds of cattle, sheep and hens, and general living conditions of the Iron Age.

A herb and medicinal garden planted as a maze (based on the Hollywood Stone in the National Museum of Ireland) is currently under construction. Also growing in it are a combination of all the plants whose seeds and husks have been found in the stomachs of the various bog bodies so far discovered, such as Tolland Man and friends from Denmark and our own Lindow Man from Cheshire (affectionately known as 'Pete Marsh').

ROYAL NAVAL HOSPITAL HASLAR

GOSPORT
HAMPSHIRE PO12 2AA

☎ TELEPHONE: 0705-584 255 EXT. 2112, COMMANDER'S
ASSISTANT

OPEN: ALTERNATIVE WEDNESDAYS BY APPOINTMENT
          ONLY.

The foundations of the RNH were laid in 1746. The architect was Theodore Jacobsen who based his design on the magnificent Foundling Hospital of Thomas Coram in London. It was intended to build eight pairs of three story blocks on the sides of a square, but when the money finally ran out the hospital was opened with only three sides of the square completed. Patients were admitted in 1763 when admissions quickly reached 2,000. Today as a District Hospital there is a ceiling of 305 with 228 beds currently manned.

The museum and library have many interesting medical historical items relating to the Navy including surgical appliances of 1923, ophthalmic lenses and spectacles of the 20th century; the foot of a 19th century Chinese woman deformed by binding; rum measures and a barrel - a practice discontinued in 1970; an amputation set; glass X-ray plates of 1923; ceramic drug jars and a leech jar; the Endean Collection of genitourinary scopes 1914-1919; the wax head of Thomas Blackman in 1845, a sailor who suffered from extensive necrosis of the bones of the cranium. Instruments from the wars include surgical instruments from the German Navy in 1944 and the contents of 2 Japanese medical chests.

There is a selection of pathology jars which are still used for teaching purposes, an illuminated display on the art of tattooing and a final room on the work of the Naval nurses at Haslar. For specific enquiries please telephone the Librarian on extension 2494.

ROYAL NAVY SUBMARINE MUSEUM

HASLAR JETTY ROAD
GOSPORT
HAMPSHIRE PO12 2AS

TELEPHONE: 0705-529 217
OPEN: MONDAY - SUNDAY ....10.00 - 4.30
          APRIL - OCTOBER
          MONDAY - SUNDAY ....10.00 - 3.30

NOVEMBER - MARCH
ADMISSION: CHARGE
SHOP. REFRESHMENTS. TOILETS.

&. DISABLED ACCESS TO GROUND FLOOR. (RING FIRST FOR
HELP TO TOP FLOOR OF MUSEUM).

Two submarines are in dry dock ready to be visited. The Holland, launched in 1901, sunk in 1912 and raised in 1982 and now fully restored. The later HMS Alliance was completed in 1947 and was in active service until 1973. A guided tour tour vividly shows how the crew of 64 lived and worked underwater. The 'Submarine Experience' is an audio-visual show which re-creates the atmosphere of being in a a submarine. The Museum has a small collection of medical items, notably a machine for measuring CO_2, apothecaries scales and stitching material from a German WW1 U-boat and the 'Keep Fit' handbook No.1.

ROYAL VICTORIA COUNTRY PARK

NETLEY ABBEY
SOUTHAMPTON
HAMPSHIRE

☽ TELEPHONE: 0703-455 157
OPEN: MONDAY - SATURDAY .... 11.00 - 5.00
        SUNDAY .... 1.00 - 5.00
        30 MARCH - 31 OCTOBER
        SUNDAY .... 10.00 - 4.00
        OCTOBER - EASTER
        MUSEUM ONLY.
        PARK OPEN AT ALL TIMES.
ADMISSION: CHARGE
SHOP. TOILETS. REFRESHMENTS AT TEA ROOMS NEARBY
IN THE PARK.

&. DISABLED ACCESS.

Situated on the shores of Southampton Water the park originally formed part of lands of Netley Abbey, the 13th century Cistercian monastry. In 1856 the first purpose-built Military Hospital was opened by Queen Victoria and Prince Albert to care for the wounded of the Crimean War. With various additions the Hospital saw service throughout the

Boer War and 1st and 2nd World Wars as one of the main centres of the Royal Army Medical Corps, until taken over by the American Forces in 1942. Today, most of the buildings have been demolished except for the Royal Chapel, now a museum. The park provides a peaceful and varied location for rallies and events, walks, barbecues and picnics, with even a narrow-guage railway on an old branch line.

The Royal Chapel and Museum shows the history of the hospital since the Crimean war. Postcards, photographs and letters from early RAMC soldiers, reconstructions of soldiers arriving wounded, a ward complete with beds, side tables and dressing packs; Queen Victoria paying one of her many visits; documentation of the USA arriving in 1943 (1/12th of all US invasion casualties were treated at Netley); WW2 preparation for D Day; Royal visits; the Army nursing service from 1863 - 1900; the Russian Navy at Netley in 1873 and a display on the life and work of Florence Nightingale.

There is a marvellous view from the top of the tower where it is possible to see Tennyson Down on the Isle of Wight. Netley is, of course, where Dr. Watson came to go through the course for surgeons in the Army in 1879 - he passed out in March 1880 - as told in 'A Study in Scarlet', the first Sherlock Holmes story.

PETERSFIELD PHYSIC GARDEN

HIGH STREET
PETERSFIELD
HAMPSHIRE

☎ TELEPHONE: 0703-268 331 (SECRETARY)
OPEN: MONDAY - SUNDAY ....9.00 - DUSK
ADMISSION: FREE - DONATIONS WELCOME
LEAFLET AVAILABLE.

♿ DISABLED ACCESS ON PATHS.

👫 PARTIES AND LECTURES BY ARRANGEMENT.

At the time of the introduction of formal physic gardens in Britain in the early 1600's, John Goodyer, one of the most eminent botanists of the period, lived and worked in

Petersfield. He grew and recorded many plants in detail and used his skill to be a 'physic' or doctor to his family and neighbours. He had an extensive library which he left on his death in 1664 to Magdalen College, Oxford.

The Hampshire Gardens Trust in 1988 received the generous gift of an ancient walled garden, one of the original 12th century burgage plots, part of which has now been laid out as a formal physic garden in the style familiar to John Goodyer. The garden also has an area with fruit trees, shrubs, old roses, wild flowers, a topiary walk and knot garden so that future generations can enjoy and conserve our heritage of plants and gardens.

The 75 medicinal plants include feverfew for headaches, primroses for 'curing the phrensie', Madonna lilies and rosemary for sweetening the breath, chamomile to be used in tea for the digestion, catmint for bruises, lovage for boils and comfrey for bleeding.

HMS VICTORY

HM NAVAL BASE
PORTSMOUTH
HAMPSHIRE PO1 3LX

☎ TELEPHONE: 0705-819 604
OPEN: MONDAY - SUNDAY .... 10.00 - 6.00
MARCH - OCTOBER
.... 10.30 - 5.30
NOVEMBER - FEBRUARY
ADMISSION: CHARGE
REFRESHMENTS. TOILETS. GUIDE BOOK AVALABLE.

&. NO DISABLED ACCESS.

👫 GROUPS BY APPOINTMENT ON 0705-839 766.
GUIDED TOURS ONLY EVERY 40 MINUITES.

In 1758 Horatio Nelson was born, son of a Norfolk parson; in the same year a First Rate Ship-of-the-Line, HMS Victory, was ordered to be built. 45 years were to pass before they finally came together, culminating in the Battle of Trafalgar on 21 October 1805. The combined fleets of France and Spain were vanquished without the loss of a single

British ship, but with the sad death of her Admiral of the Fleet, Lord Nelson. The orlop deck, below the gundeck, became the operating theatre and hospital in battle and it is here that Nelson died. The dispensary has a display of scalpels, saws, forceps, teeth extractors, sounds, fleams, a small medicine chest and apothecaries jars, the red paint disguising the blood that was spilt during the operations.

MARY ROSE

HM NAVAL BASE
PORTSMOUTH
HAMPSHIRE PO1 3LX

① TELEPHONE: 0705-750 521
OPEN: MONDAY - SUNDAY ....10.00 - 7.00
       JULY & AUGUST
       ....10.00 - 5.30
       MARCH - OCTOBER
       ....10.30 - 5.00
       NOVEMBER - FEBRUARY
       LAST TOUR 1 HOUR BEFORE CLOSING
ADMISSION: CHARGE
SHOP. REFRESHMENTS. TOILETS.
& DISABLED ACCESS TO ALL EXHIBITS (BOOK IN ADVANCE).

Amidst much publicity and excitement the Mary Rose, Tudor warship of Henry VIII, which had sunk a mile and a quarter from the entrance to Portsmouth harbour in 1545, was finally brought to the surface on 11th Ocotober 1982. The remains of the solid oak hull, carefully preserved in a dry dock, constantly sprayed with recycled chilled water in an atmosphere of 95% humidity, is an awe-inspiring sight, standing as high as a four-storey building. Marked by a pole is the barber surgeon's cabin, an area of 6 square yards with only 5'6" headroom. The artefacts recovered from the ship are well displayed in the adjoining museum. Pewter plates tankards and spoons; candleholders of pewter, brass and wood; tabor pipes and a drum; dice and an elaborate gaming board; book covers, quill pens and inkwells; and a selection of items that were used to 'make do and mend'. A large wooden chest was recovered from the barber surgeon's cabin which contained 64 objects, including 9 wooden lidded canisters of ointments and a similar one with peppercorns - (used for ague and quinsy). 3 metal syringes for urethral injections and the handles of surgical tools, cauteries, razors, whetstones, a brass shaving bowl and 5 corked flagons which may have been imported as medical containers. Also on display are guns, archery equipment and munitions of war.

ROYAL NAVAL MUSEUM

HM NAVAL BASE
PORTSMOUTH
HAMPSHIRE PO1 3LX

✆ TELEPHONE: 0705-733 060
OPEN: MONDAY - SUNDAY .... 10.30 - 5.00
SUBJECT TO ALTERATION DUE TO MANPOWER RESTRICTIONS.
ADMISSION: CHARGE
SHOP. REFRESHMENTS. TOILETS.

♿ DISABLED ACCESS.

GROUPS BY APPOINTMENT ON 0705-839 766.

The museum stands in the centre of Portsmouth's historic Naval Base. It has 5 large galleries packed with mementoes of those who have served their country at sea through a thousand years of peace and war. Throughout the museum are references to the life and work of the ship's doctor. A leech jar of 1800, a picture of Dr. William Beatty's dispensary on IIMS Victory, the dispensary on HMS Melbourne, a medal of Assistant Surgeon Andrew Daly awarded after the capture of the French ships Marengo and Belle Pouce off Brest. A picture of the sick bay on HMS Hannibal 1896, and the hospital ship used in the Crimean War in 1854.

TUDOR HOUSE MUSEUM

BUGLE STREET
SOUTHAMPTON
HAMPSHIRE

☎ TELEPHONE: 0703-332 513
OPEN: TUESDAY - FRIDAY .... 10.00 - 12.00 & 1.00 - 5.00
          SATURDAY .... 1.00 - 12.00 & 1.00 - 4.00
          SUNDAY .... 2.00 - 5.00
ADMISSION: FREE
SHOP. TOILETS.

&. DISABLED ACCESS TO GROUND FLOOR AND GARDENS.

Situated in the 'Old Town', Tudor House was built towards the end of the 15th century for Sir John Dawtrey, a merchant and Controller of Customs (the house is close to the Waterfront). The Great Hall, central to Tudor life, has furniture and fittings of that period. The kitchen and upstairs rooms show Victorian and Edwardian domestic and social artefacts including some medical items. These are a china slipper bedpan, pill rolling equipment, dental tools, false teeth of porcelain, a scarifier, ivory tooth picks, bottles and lids of patent medicines and a metal syringe. In a cabinet of pottery is an 18th century mortar and an apothecary's jar. A further dispaly shows a varied collection of 18th and 19th century spectacles.

The Tudor Garden is an exquisite example of a 'living museum' in which small samples of large features can be fully maintained in detail and small numbers of correct plants can be grown. The features include a secret garden, fountain plot, heraldic ornaments, arbour, orchard, parapet and mount, close walks, quarters or square beds, knots, hedges and topiary and a herb garden. The latter has hyssop for the cure of a cough, juniper to be burned in times of plague, borage to make the mind glad, artemesia to rid oneself of fleas and oregano for digestion, amongst many others. Most of the plants by their name, colour or use were symbolic and an excellent descriptive booklet is available.

ROYAL MARINE MUSEUM

ROYAL MARINES EASTNEY
SOUTHSEA
HAMPSHIRE P04 9PX

TELEPHONE: 0705-819 385
OPEN: MONDAY - SUNDAY .... 10.00 - 5.30
          EASTER - SEPTEMBER 30TH
          .... 10.00 - 4.30
          OCTOBER - MARCH
ADMISSION: CHARGE
SHOP. REFRESHMENTS. TOILETS.

NO DISABLED ACCESS (STAIRS TO ENTRANCE).

GROUPS BY APPOINTMENT FOR GUIDED TOURS.

The Royal Marines were raised in 1664 as 'sea soldiers' and the museum has a wide range of objects, books, documents, pictures and photographs relating to thier history. The archives have a historical photographic collection and reference library available to the public for research purposes. The medical items include a 1750's syringe, a WW1 general surgical kit, personal medical kits issued to those Marines serving in the tropics and guide lines for service men going to the Far East. Further material is available by appointment.

WINCHESTER CITY MUSEUM

THE SQUARE
WINCHESTER
HAMPSHIRE

TELEPHONE: 0962-863 064
OPEN: MONDAY - SATURDAY .... 10.00 - 5.00
          SUNDAY .... 2.00 - 5.00
          APRIL - SEPTEMBER
          TUESDAY - SATURDAY .... 10.00 - 5.00
          SUNDAY .... 2.00 - 4.00
          OCTOBER - MARCH
ADMISSION: FREE
SHOP.

DISABLED ACCESS TO GROUND FLOOR.

The archaeology and history of Winchester and the surrounding countryside have produced a wide and varying collection of Roman, Anglo-Saxon, and medieval artefacts, including metalwork, sculpture, glass, ceramics and jewellery. The reconstructed 19th century shops show a local tobacconist, butcher and the pharmacy of Richard Hunt. Hunt's unique collection of pharmaceutical furnishings ranges from the 18th to the 20th centuries with some early Delftware jars and green painted dry drug drawers each with a painted scroll bearing the name of the contents in black Roman lettering. There are also the original mahogany counter panels, undecorated 19th century drawers and glass doors leading to the preparation room behind, showing pill making equipment and recipe and prescription books.

Hereford & Worcester

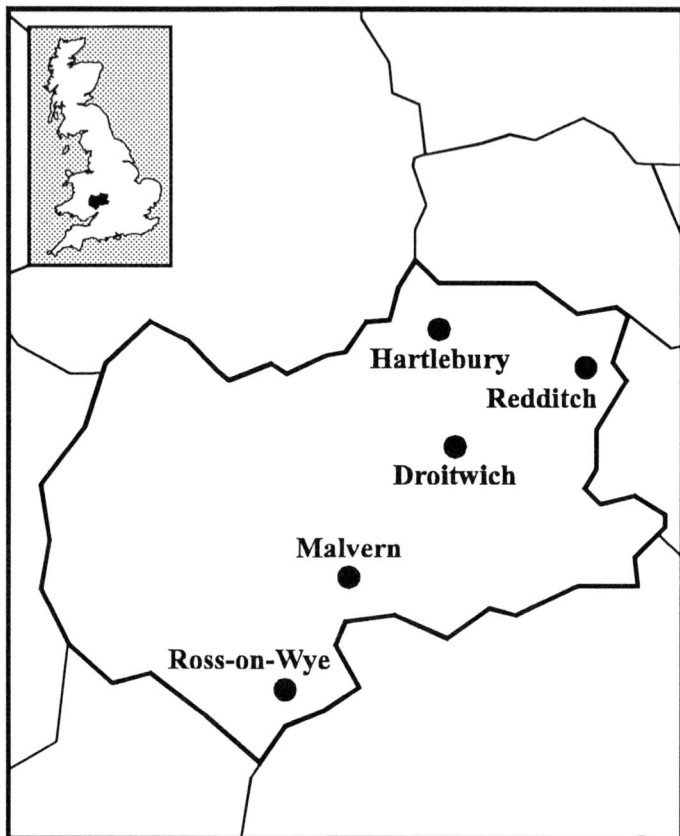

DROITWICH HERITAGE CENTRE

ST. RICHARDS HOUSE
VICTORIA SQUARE
DROITWICH
HEREFORD & WORCESTER WR9 8DS

TELEPHONE: 0905-774 312
OPEN: MONDAY - FRIDAY ....9.00 - 5.00
SATURDAY...10.00 - 4.00
APRIL - OCTOBER
MONDAY - FRIDAY ....9.00 - 4.30
SATURDAY...10.00 - 4.00

NOVEMBER - MARCH
ADMISSION: FREE
SHOP. MEN'S TOILET.

  ♿   DISABLED ACCESS TO ALL MUSEUM.

Salt has been produced in Droitwich for over 2,000 years and the Heritage Centre reflects the town's development from the early Iron-age to a fashionable 19th century spa town. In 1830 the first Brine Baths were built which brought relief to many, including a few miraculous cures, notably cholera! A skeleton in the museum is 1,800 years old and was found in a brine pit complete with teeth. Other items include salt-making barrels and equipment, and bath chairs.

Visitors do not drink the brine - containing 2 1/2 pounds of salt per gallon of water - but experience the therapeutic and remedial benefits of floating weightless in the warm brine of the bathing pool in St. Andrew's road, on the site of the original historic Spa baths. (Open to the public Monday - Friday, 12.00 - 8.00pm; Saturday, 10.00 - 5.00; Sunday, 10.00 - 4.00; book in advance on 0905-794 894.)

HEREFORD & WORCESTER COUNTY MUSEUM

HARTLEBURY CASTLE
HARTLEBURY
Nr. KIDDERMINSTER
HEREFORD & WORCESTER DY11 7XZ

☎ TELEPHONE: 0299-250 416/250 560
OPEN: MONDAY - THURSDAY ....10.00 - 5.00
FRIDAY & SUNDAY ....2.00 - 5.00
B.H. ....10.00 - 5.00
CLOSED: GOOD FRIDAY & SATURDAY
1ST MARCH - 30TH NOVEMBER
ADMISSION: CHARGE
TOILETS. REFRESHMENTS. SHOP. PICNIC AREA.
EDUCATION SERVICE.

  ♿   DISABLED ACCESS GROUND FLOOR ONLY.

  🚶   PARTIES BY APPOINTMENT.

The museum is housed in the north wing of Hartlebury Castle the Bishop of Worcester's official residence. The manor was given to the Bishops in 850 and became a fortified manor surrounded by a moat, but from the 17th century was embellished in the style of a country gentleman's residence. Opened in 1966 the Museum's objective was to "illustrate the broad basis of the life of Worcestershire people through the centuries". To this end there is a display of agricultural bygones, aspects of measurement, costumes and textiles, a glass room, children's gallery, a Georgian room and Victorian drawing room. A display of mahogany medicine chests, surgical cases, fleams, cupping sets, apothecary's scales, pill boxes, early 20th century hearing aid, a 19th century stethoscope, a late 18th century gruel warmer and some medical text books. A small reserve collection is available by appointment and includes some medical instruments.

MALVERN HILLS MUSEUM

THE ABBEY GATEWAY
ABBEY ROAD
MALVERN
HEREFORD & WORCESTER WR14 3HG

☎ TELEPHONE: 0684-567 811
    OPEN: MONDAY - SUNDAY .... 10.30 - 5.00
              CLOSED WEDNESDAY
              MID MAY - END OCTOBER
    ADMISSION: CHARGE
    SHOP.
♿ NO DISABLED ACCESS.

Popular in the mid 19th century when is was fashionable to take the 'water cure' Malvern became one of the foremost spas. Not because the waters contained an excessive mineral content but because of their lack of it and for their great purity.

A small museum in the Abbey gateway traces the success of this 'water cure' together with the historical associations of Elgar and Shaw.

FORGE MILL NEEDLE MUSEUM

NEEDLE MILL LANE
RIVERSIDE
REDDITCH
WORCESTERSHIRE B97 6RR

☾ TELEPHONE: 0527-62509
OPEN: MONDAY - THURSDAY ....11.00 - 4.30
        SATURDAY...2.00 - 5.00
        SUNDAY & B.H. ....1.00 - 5.00
        1ST MARCH - 31 OCTOBER
        NOVEMBER: MONDAY- THURSDAY
CLOSED: DECEMBER
ADMISSION: CHARGE TO NEEDLE MUSEUM & VISITOR
CENTRE AT BORDERSLEY ABBEY
SHOP. REFRESHMENTS. TOILETS.

&. DISABLED ACCESS TO GROUND FLOOR.

⅍ GUIDED TOURS BY ARRANGEMENT.

The Museum, opened by the Queen in 1983, preserves items from the once world-famous Redditch needle and fishing tackle industries. It is housed in a former 18th century needle scouring (polishing) mill with much of the original machinery restored to working order, powered by one of the few working water wheels in the West Midlands.

There are 10 sample books of surgeon's needles that date from 1900-1950, some of which are on display and others available to view by appointment. All are in superb condition. Various surgical needle catalogues, printing blocks for surgical needle packets and catalogues and a wide variety of the dies used for making the surgical needles (these can be viewed by request) are on display together with modern hypodermic and surgical needles from local factories.

Other displays show some of the more unusual needles from beading, bookbinding and sailmaking to smocking, with examples of old crafts and pastimes. Also the world's smallest and largest needle and one of the oldest types, 'Eve's needle'.

Adjacent to the Museum are the remains of the 12th century Cistercian Bordesley Abbey whose excavated finds are displayed in the Visitor Centre.

THE LOST STREET MUSEUM

PALMA COURT
27 BROOKEND STREET
ROSS-ON-WYE
HEREFORD & WORCESTER

① TELEPHONE: 0989 62752
OPEN: MONDAY - SATURDAY .... 10.00 - 5.00
            SUNDAY .... 11.00 - 5.00
TOILETS. REFRESHMENTS IN COURTYARD.
& NO DISABLED ACCESS.

In a courtyard behind the main street is a time capsule of shops and a pub dating from 1885 - 1935. Each shop has an original front and interior and is stocked with items in keeping with its period. The tobacconist's is crowded with cigarette and chocolate vending machines and a collection of matchboxes. A ladies outfitters evokes an era of elegance, and the music shop has both gramophones and phonographs. The grocer's and toy shops, glass, motorcycle and chemist shops give an insight into the delights of shopping in the past. The chemist's shop has bottles, pills, potions and ointments, many with original labels and packaging.

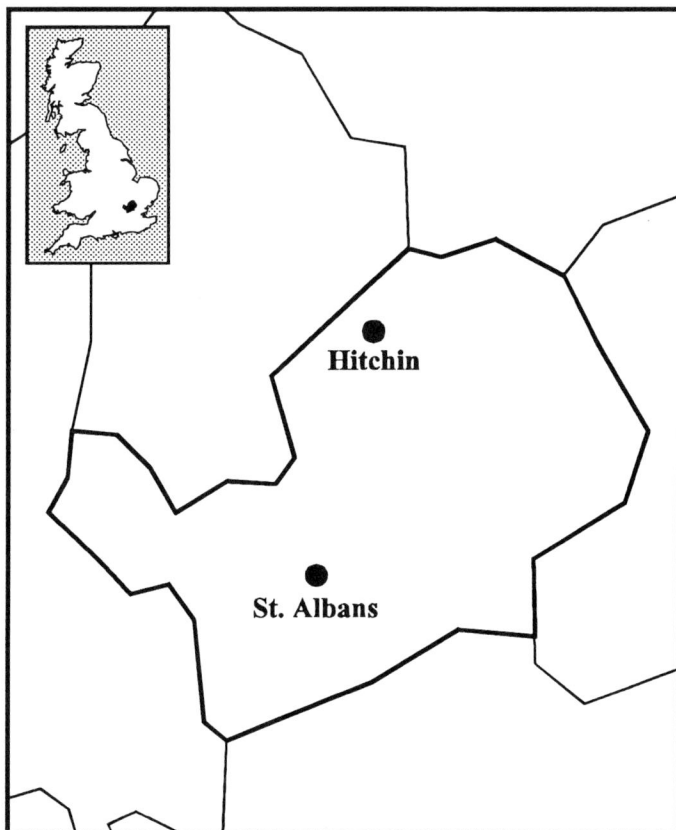

HITCHIN MUSEUM

PAYNES PARK
HITCHIN
HERTFORDSHIRE

ⓓ TELEPHONE: 0462-434 476
  OPEN: MONDAY - SATURDAY.................................10.00 - 5.00
      EXCEPT PUBLIC HOLIDAYS
      SUNDAY..2.00 - 4.30
  ADMISSION: FREE
  SHOP.
♿ DISABLED ACCESS TO GROUND FLOOR ONLY.

Housing displays on local industries and domestic life with a major collection of historical costume and material belonging to the Hertfordshire Yeomanry Trust, the museum is unique in combining a physic garden and chemist's shop reflecting the modern and historical importance of medicinal plants. The Victorian chemist's shop contains a wide range of pills, potions, ointments, bottles and jars. On one side of the shop is a display of lavender products manufactured by Perks Llewellyn - at one time Hitchin was a major producer of lavender in the country. The Physic Garden has been divided into categories according to usage, ie: internal and external ailments, household dyes and household and culinary uses. The William Ransom borders grow some of the plants originally used by this first chemist in Hitchin (1846). Joseph Lister came to be educated in Hitchin as a boy of 11 and the museum holds some of his original anatomical drawings and anatomical instruments. A folder of reference is available for serious researchers by prior appointment.

MUSEUM OF ST. ALBANS

HATFIELD ROAD
ST. ALBANS
HERTFORDSHIRE AL1 3RS

☎ TELEPHONE: 0727-56679
OPEN: MONDAY - SATURDAY .... 10.00 - 5.00
              SUNDAY .... 2.00 - 5.00
ADMISSION: CHARGE, FREE TO LOCAL RESIDENTS
SHOP. TOILETS.

&. DISABLED ACCESS TO GROUND FLOOR.

The 'Story of St. Albans' from the departure of the Romans to the present day includes a collection of apothecary's equipment, surgeon's and dental instruments and a gallery on public health. This shows a typical Victorian laundry day with an old tin bath and various domestic utilities for keeping clean. The newest gallery shows the vast Salaman collection of craft tools many of which belonged to woodworkers and turners.

Further medical items are held in the reserve collection and are available to view by appointment only on application to the keeper of Social History.

THE VERULAMIUM MUSEUM

ST. MICHAELS
ST. ALBANS
HERTFORDSHIRE AL3 4SW

℡ TELEPHONE: 0727-819 339
OPEN: MONDAY - SATURDAY.................................10.00 - 5.30
              LAST ADMISSION 5.00
              SUNDAY...2.00 - 5.00
ADMISSION: CHARGE
SHOP. TOILETS IN CAR PARK.
♿ DISABLED ACCESS.

Standing on the site of the Roman City of Verulamium the excavated artefacts include some of the best examples of mosaics in the country. Items of Roman medical equipment is also on display and includes a copy of an oculist's stamp, bronze forceps, a bronze probe with a twisted handle, possible bronze surgical instruments from 75-105 A.D. and a bronze scalpel from 225-250 A.D.

Humberside

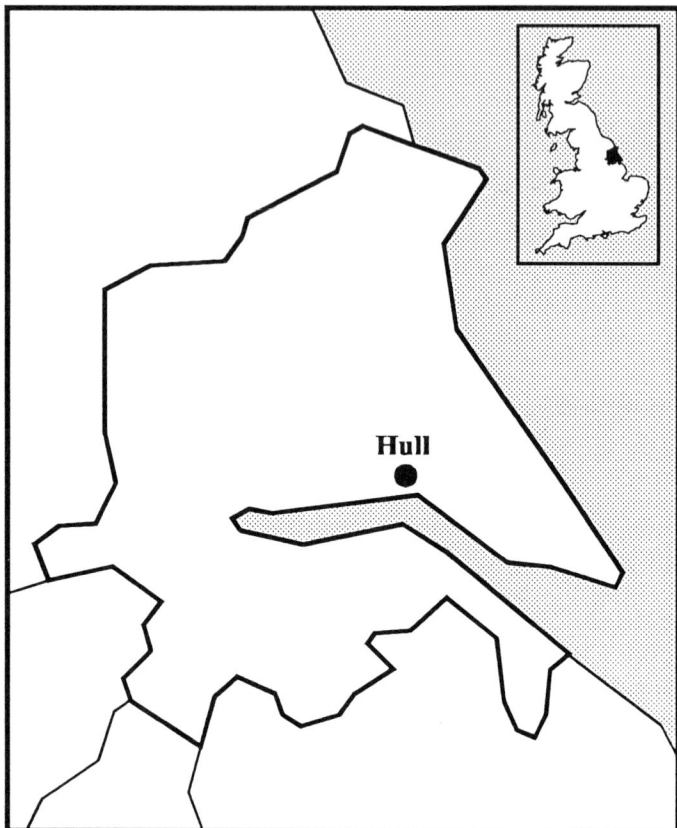

WILBERFORCE HOUSE & GEORGIAN HOUSES

23 - 25 HIGH STREET
HULL
HUMBERSIDE

TELEPHONE: 0482-593 921
OPEN: MONDAY - SATURDAY .... 10.00 - 5.00
              SUNDAY .... 1.30 - 4.30
ADMISSION: FREE
SHOP. TOILETS.

DISABLED ACCESS TO GROUND FLOOR ONLY.

The museum is in several 17th and 18th century merchant's houses, one of which was the home of William Wilberforce, the slave emancipator, and contains exhibitions relating to his fight against slavery. There are interesting collections of costumes, dolls, furniture and silver. The chemist's shop is a reconstruction of Castlelow's Pharmacy of Leeds. Mr. Walter Castlelow took over the practice in 1907 and worked until his death in 1974, aged 98, when he was apparently the oldest practising pharmacist in the country. The mahogany interior fittings consist of a counter with a screened dispensing area; a drug run; shelves and glass fronted cabinets, many from the original shop (1841). The pharmacy contains hundreds of liquids and powders in their original glass rounds, packets and bottles of pills, some made up by Mr. Castlelow himself. Other items include make-up, nivea products, stocking dye, toiletries, mousetraps and perfume bottles. (Information from Wilberforce House Museum, Hull City Museums & Art Galleries, Hull City Council.)

Kent

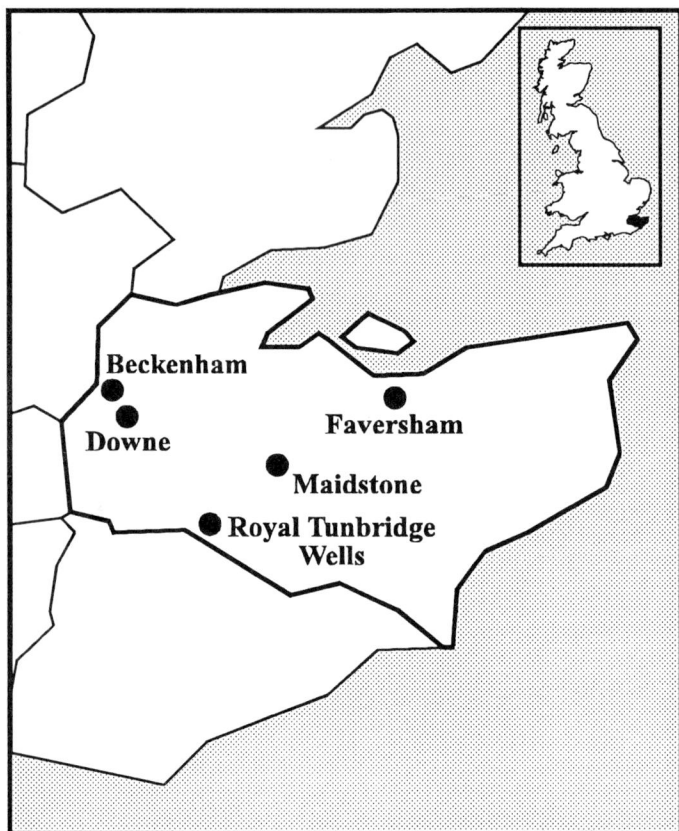

BETHLEM ROYAL HOSPITAL ARCHIVES & MUSEUM

THE BETHLEM ROYAL HOSPITAL
MONKS ORCHARD ROAD
BECKENHAM
KENT BR3 3BX

℡ TELEPHONE: 081-777 6611 EXT. 4307
    OPEN: MONDAY - FRIDAY .... 9.30 - 5.30
                BY APPOINTMENT ONLY
    ADMISSION: FREE

♿ DISABLED ACCESS DIFFICULT.

The Bethlem Royal Hospital and the Maudsley Hospital is a postgraduate psychiatric teaching hospital and a leading centre for research in psychiatry. It was formed in 1948 by the union of the Bethlem Hospital (the original 'Bedlam') and the Maudsley (a London County Council Mental Hospital).

Objects in the museum include the huge sculptures by Cibber of Madness and Melancholy from the gates of the 17th century Bedlam and a small amount of historical material. The largest and most exciting display in the museum concentrates on the paintings of artists who have suffered from mental disorder. There are 13 watercolours by the Victorian artist Richard Dadd, paintings by Jonathan Martin and over 200 examples of works by psychiatric patients who were at Bethlem when Sir. T. B. Hyslop was medical superintendent.

In 1986 the museum acquired the Guttmann-Maclay Collection from the Institute of Psychiatry. These include works by Louis Wain, Nijinsky and William Kurelek.

THE CHARLES DARWIN MEMORIAL MUSEUM

DOWN HOUSE
LUXTED ROAD
DOWNE
KENT BN6 7JT

℡ TELEPHONE: 0689-859 119
OPEN: WEDNESDAYS - SUNDAYS............................1.00 - 6.00
              & B.H. MON.
              MARCH - DECEMBER 15th.
ADMISSION: CHARGE
SHOP. TOILETS.

Charles Robert Darwin was born in Shrewsbury on 12th February 1809 and died at Down House on 19th April 1882. His bronze statue sits in front of the former Shrewsbury school buildings in Castle Street. In 1825 Charles joined his brother at Edinburgh to study medicine but this was unsuccessful so he was sent to Christ's College Cambridge to train for the church. He gained his B.A. and made friends with the Professor of Botany, John Stephen Henslow. It was

Henslow who in 1831 secured him a place on Captain Robert Fitzroy's ship HMS Beagle. Their object was to make a survey of the South American coast. The voyage took almost five years and even before his return his name was known in scientific circles for the specimens he sent home. On 27th January 1839 he married his first cousin Emma Wedgwood and they lived in Upper Gower Street (Blue Plaque); three years later they moved with their two children to Downe in Kent. His publications over the ensuing years ensured his name was well known by the time The Origin Of The Species By Natural Selection was published in 1859. His final years were full of happiness and prosperity and he and Emma and their surviving seven children lived in an atmosphere of great affection.

The house has been preserved as a national memorial by a distinguished London surgeon, Sir George Buckston Browne, who provided the necessary funds and opened it to the public in 1929. Towards the end of 1952 the property was offered to and accepted by the Royal College of Surgeons which has now assumed the task of maintaining Charles Darwin's home as a memorial. The rooms open to the public are on the ground floor. The Old Study where most of Darwin's work was done is decorated and furnished almost as he knew it. The drawing room has been restored and the former dining-room devoted to Darwin's journey on the Beagle. The works belonging to his grandfather, the physician Erasmus Darwin, are also on display. Outside the garden remains much as Darwin knew it and you may still follow in his footsteps along the 'thinking path' and through the sand-walk wood.

FLEUR DE LIS HERITAGE CENTRE

PRESTON STREET
FAVERSHAM
KENT ME13 8NS

ⓓ TELEPHONE: 0795-534 542
OPEN: MONDAY - SATURDAY .... 9.30 - 1.00 & 2.00 - 4.00
               EASTER TO END SEPTEMBER 4.30
CLOSED: THURSDAY & B.H.

ADMISSION: CHARGE
SHOP.

In one of Britain's finest heritage towns the Centre, in a 15th century building, illustrates how the town has evolved over more than 1,000 years. Vividly brought to life are award winning displays on breweries, brickfields, explosives, hop picking, shipbuilding, fire services, schools and hospitals. The history of the local Cottage Hospital is displayed together with some medical instruments and a hand-pushed ambulance.

COBTREE MUSEUM OF KENT LIFE

LOCK LANE
SANDLING
MAIDSTONE
KENT ME14 3AU

TELEPHONE: 0622-763 936
OPEN: MONDAY - SUNDAY ....11.00 - 6.00
                EASTER - OCTOBER
                SUNDAY..11.00 - 5.00
                NOVEMBER - MARCH
ADMISSION: CHARGE
SHOP. REFRESHMENTS. TOILETS. PICNIC AREA. CRAFT
FAIRS & SPECIAL EVENTS.

DISABLED ACCESS TO WHOLE SITE.

Set in 27 acres of rural landscape overlooking the River Medway, the museum tells the story of the Kent countryside from hops and fruit to agricultural machinery and livestock. Displays are housed in the 18th century barn and oast house and the row of reconstructed hoppers' huts creates a feeling of rural life through the ages in the 'Garden of England'.

Other attractions on the site include a working hop garden, orchard, herb garden, market garden and livestock. Craft demonstrations take place on selected Sundays of spinning, blacksmithing, bee-keeping, rush and cane work and other skills.

The herb garden has many medicinal plants and a board explains their uses:- garlic for protection against colds, worms, dysentery and fever; orris for bronchitis, diarrhoea and dropsy; yarrow whose young leaves aid toothache; hyssop to aid digestion of fatty fish and meat; rue for hysteria, epilepsy, blood pressure, rheumatism and arthritis; marigold as an antiseptic and as an excellent skin healer for cracked skin and chapped lips; elecampane whose candied roots were sucked to alleviate asthma and indigestion; betony for jaundice, gout, convulsions, dropsy and head troubles; liquorice for coughs, bronchitis and gastric ulcers; agrimony often regarded as a heal all but good for gastrointestinal complaints and loosestrife for checking bleeding of the mouth, nose and wounds.

A DAY AT THE WELLS

THE CORN EXCHANGE
THE PANTILES
ROYAL TUNBRIDGE WELLS
KENT TN2 5QJ

☏ TELEPHONE: 0892-546 545
OPEN: MONDAY - SUNDAY .... 9.30 - 5.30
           APRIL - OCTOBER
           MONDAY - SUNDAY .... 10.00 - 4.00
           NOVEMBER - MARCH
SHOP. TOILETS.
♿ DISABLED ACCESS BOOK IN ADVANCE.

The origins of the spa go back to the 18th century when Lord North claimed that a spring had cured a 'lingering comsumptive disorder'. The Chalybeate spring, in the Pantiles, can still be tasted on a summer afternoon, served by the 'dipper'.

A Day At The Wells recreates life in the 18th century at a time of elegance and scandal with the sights, sounds and smells of Georgian England when Beau Nash was the arbiter of gentility and good taste.

Lancashire

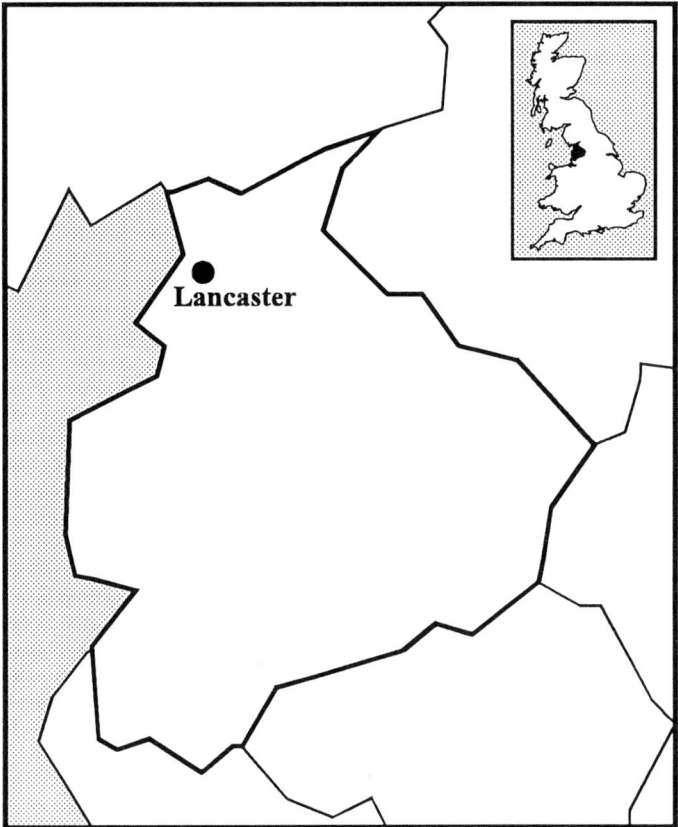

THE CITY MUSEUM

MARKET SQUARE
LANCASTER
LANCASHIRE LA1 1HT

☎ TELEPHONE: 0524-64637
OPEN: MONDAY - SATURDAY..................................10.00 - 5.00
ADMISSION: FREE
SHOP.

♿ DISABLED ACCESS TO GROUND FLOOR ONLY.

Housed in the old Town Hall of 1783 the museum traces the history of the surrounding area from archaeological finds to local industries. These include clog-making, pottery, textiles, linoleum and cabinet-making. Amongst the miscellaneous medical items are some midwifery equipment, domestic medicine bottles and pill boxes. The comprehensive collection of spectacles is available to view by appointment only. The local mental hospital is hoping to set up its own museum at a future date.

Leicestershire

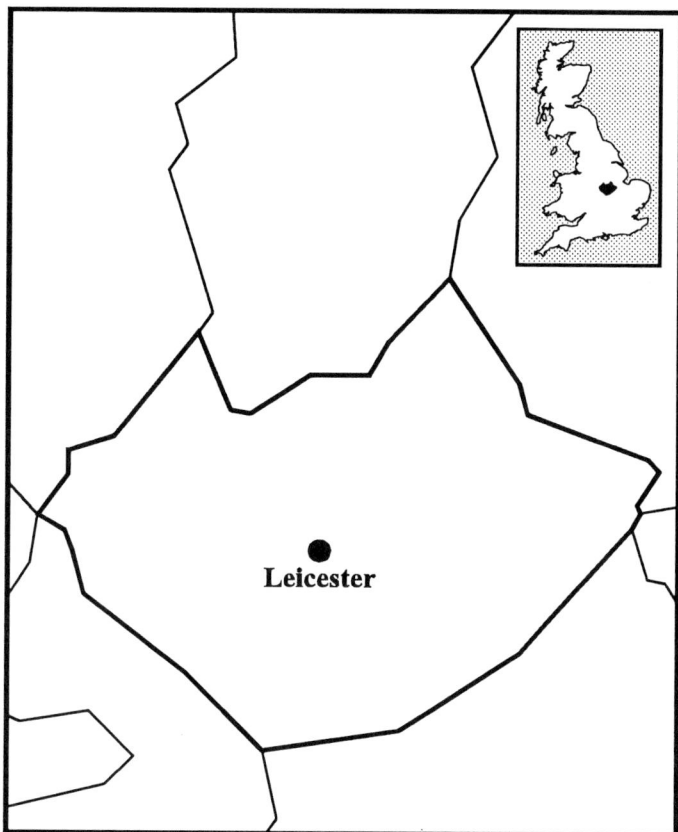

NEWARKE HOUSES MUSEUM

THE NEWARKE
LEICESTER
LEICESTERSHIRE LE2 7BY

TELEPHONE: 0533-554 100
OPEN: MONDAY - SATURDAY.................................10.00 - 5.30
                SUNDAY...2.00 - 5.30
ADMISSION: FREE
SHOP.

DISABLED ACCESS TO GOUND FLOOR.

Two separate 16th century houses have combined to provide an authentic setting to show the social history of Leicestershire during the last 500 years. There are galleries of domestic life, toys, coins and hygiene. The latter (popularly known as the 'loo room') has a number of lavishly decorated Victorian toilets. A chemist's dispensary of the early 1930's has been reconstructed which, besides the usual pill making equipment, has some medical equipment and instruments. Perhaps the most famous exhibit is Daniel Lambert, Leicestershire's fat man. He was born in 1770 and took over his father's job as keeper of the prison in 1793 by which time his weight has increased to 32 stones. In 1805 when the prison closed he decided to exhibit himself in London. He was a very witty but dignified man and people liked to come to converse with him as well as to stare. In 1809 he went to the races at Stamford in Lincolnshire but died suddenly at the Waggon and Horses Inn. His death was probably due to disease since he did not overeat or drink. His height was 5'11", waist 9'4", calf 3'1", weight 52 stones; a full size life model with his clothes, chair and paintings are in a special gallery. A street scene of the 1800's, period garden and exhibition gallery complete this charming museum. The Library has several catalogues of medical equipment and files on local hospitals which may be seen by appointment.

ROYAL INFIRMARY HISTORY MUSEUM

        KNIGHTON STREET NURSES HOME
        ROYAL INFIRMARY
        LEICESTER
        LEICESTERSHIRE

① TELEPHONE: 0533-541 414
        OPEN: TUESDAY & WEDNESDAY ....12.00 - 2.00
        ADMISSION: FREE
        OTHER TIMES BY APPOINTMENT ON 085883 523
        HISTORY BOOK ON SALE.
& DISABLED ACCESS.

The museum contains displays of the written and pictorial history of the Leicester Royal Infirmary from its origin in 1771 to 1980. A collection of medical and surgical equipment, fleams and lances, stethoscopes, amputation sets, instruments, anaesthetic memorabilia and domestic medical chests, chart the history of medicine through the years. Archive material of various departments is also available.

Lincolnshire

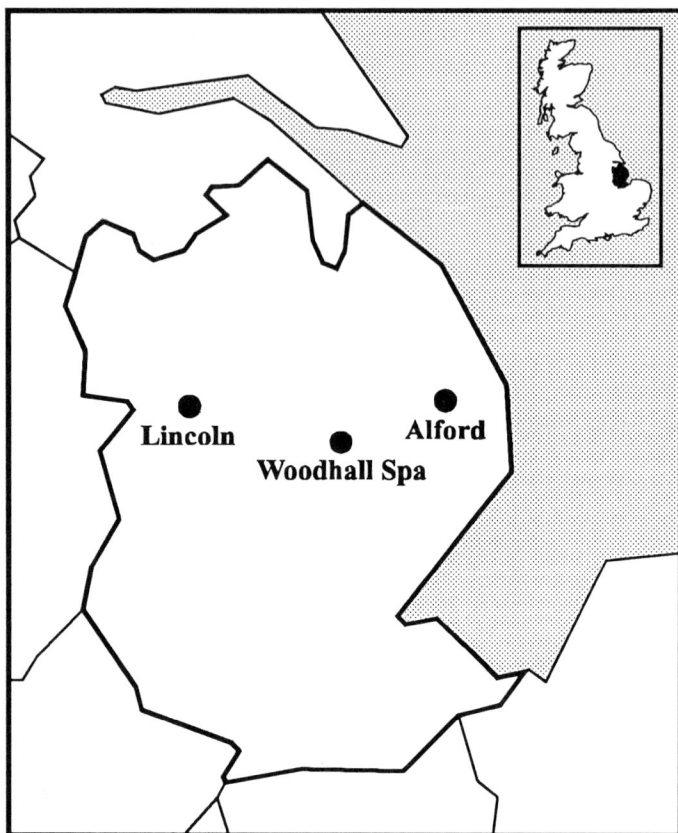

ALFORD MANOR HOUSE FOLK MUSEUM

WEST STREET
ALFORD
LINCOLNSHIRE LN13 9DJ

TELEPHONE: 0507-466 488
OPEN: MONDAY - SATURDAY .... 10.30 - 4.30
         SUNDAY .... 1.00 - 4.30
         EARLY MAY - EARLY OCTOBER
ADMISSION: CHARGE
REFRESHMENTS (BY ARRANGEMENT). TOILETS.

DISABLED ACCESS TO GROUND FLOOR LIMITED.

The building is unusual in that it is a thatched manor house dating from 1630. It was bequeathed to the Alford Civic Trust in 1967, opened as a folk museum two years later and is now maintained by volunteers of the Civic Trust.

The local history room shows a model of a long barrow and pans used in the production of salt from the sea water together with examples of local crafts and trades. The kitchen has equipment used by J. Hildred in his confectionery business in 1838, whilst the dairy has canning and sealing equipment used by members of the W.V.S. for the storage of home-produced fruit and vegetables. A police cell, boot and shoe maker, schoolroom, maid's room and nursery, a veterinary display and a chemist's shop provide an interesting collection of memorabilia. The chemist's shop comes from 2 old local shops which served the town and surrounding area making their own pills, potions and purges. Many of their well-tried prescriptions and remedies are recorded in the books exhibited. Also on display are Red Cross and other medical artefacts.

The Alford Anglo-American Exhibition stresses the connection with Captain John Smith, Anne Hutchinson (both locally born) and Thomas Paine, who spent only a short time in Alford.

MUSEUM OF LINCOLNSHIRE LIFE

BURTON ROAD
LINCOLN
LINCOLNSHIRE LN1 3LY

ⓘ TELEPHONE: 0522-528 448
OPEN: MONDAY - SUNDAY ....10.00 - 5.30
MAY - SEPTEMBER
MONDAY - SATURDAY................................10.00 - 5.30
SUNDAY...2.00 - 5.30,
OCTOBER - APRIL
ADMISSION: CHARGE
SHOP. REFRESHMENTS. TOILETS.

 ♿ DISABLED ACCESS TO GROUND FLOOR.

 ♟ EVENING PARTY VISITS BY ARRANGEMENT.

The building which the museum occupies was once the headquarters of the Royal North Lincoln Militia, built in 1857. Known as 'The Old Barracks' the museum represents the fens, farming, folk life and factory production of the surrounding area. There are displays of community life with a school, chapel, barracks and parish hall, pub and police station and a wing illustrating the rooms of an Edwardian house. Several large exhibits include the Royal Lincolnshire Regiment, an agricultural and industry gallery, and 'Commercial Row'. In this there is a chemist's shop of 1890/1900 complete with mahogany drug run, bottles and jars, inhaler, tincture press, weighing scales, prescription books, an artificial arm and wooden peg leg, glass syringe and an Army and Navy paper cover for the seat of a lavatory! Apparatus for reviving the drowned can be seen by appointment.

WOODHALL SPA COTTAGE MUSEUM

THE BUNGALOW
IDDESLEIGH ROAD
WOODHALL SPA
LINCOLNSHIRE LN10 6SH

℗ TELEPHONE: 0526-52955
OPEN: MONDAY - SUNDAY .... 10.00 - 5.00
EASTER - SEPTEMBER
ADMISSION: CHARGE
SHOP.
& DISABLED ACCESS DIFFICULT.

The Spa owes its origins to John Parkinson of Bolingbroke whose 3 dreams were to plant a forest, build a city and sink a coal mine. In 1821 he started to sink a shaft but after various disasters it flooded and overflowed into a surrounding ditch. Legend says cattle drinking from the ditch were cured of ailments. Local inhabitants found the water relieved the symptoms of rheumatism, gout and scurvy. Thomas Hotchkin, Lord of the Manor, purchased the land, found the water contained six times more iodine and bromine than any known mineral water, and in 1839 built the first Pump room and Bath House and the Victoria Hotel. People came by train to take the water, mud baths and various other treatments.

The museum and Visitor Centre is housed in a bungalow erected in 1887 which was the home of Thomas Wield and his family. From the 1890's he made donkey-drawn bath chairs while his son developed a flair for making precision instruments, including grinding lenses and cameras. At his death in 1965 he left a large collection of photographs, recording the events and people in the history of the spa from 1889-1920, which are on display in the museum.

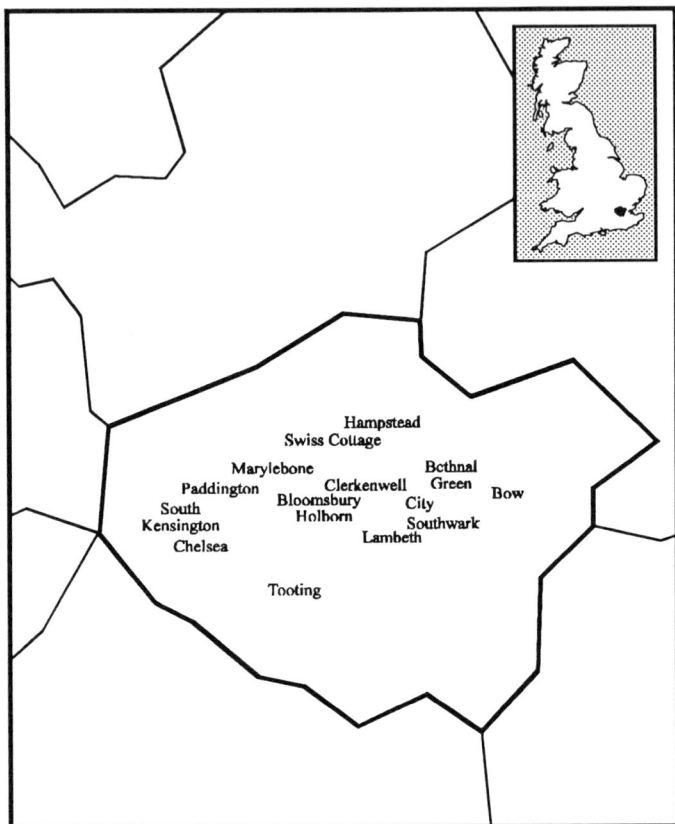

B.O.C. (British Oxygen Company) MUSEUM

THE ASSOCIATION OF ANAESTHETISTS OF GREAT BRITAIN
AND IRELAND
9 BEDFORD SQUARE
LONDON WC1B 3RA

☎ TELEPHONE: 071-631 1650
OPEN: BY APPOINTMENT ONLY, FOR RESEARCH

The only complete Georgian Square left in Bloomsbury with many of the original fixtures and fittings, No. 9 has an elegant door way complete with 'link snuffer'. In the lower ground floor is the unique Charles King Collection of historic anaesthetic apparatus.

BRITISH DENTAL ASSOCIATION MUSEUM

64 WIMPOLE STREET
LONDON W1M 8AL

℡ TELEPHONE: 071-935 0875 EXT. 209
OPEN: MONDAY - FRIDAY ....9.00 - 5.00
ADMISSION: FREE

♿ DISABLED ACCESS, RING FIRST.

In 1919 the British Dental Association moved to new headquarters in Russell Square and established a library in the care of Lilian Lindsay, the first woman to qualify as a dentist in Britain. Many books, instruments and surgery equipment were donated then and over the years so that even the new headquarters in Wimpole Street are not adequate in size to hold the large collection.

In the lower gallery of the museum is a reconstructed surgery of 1860 with furniture from the practice of John Tomes, who was a founder member and the first President of the British Dental Association. The other surgery dates from 1899, after the 1878 Dentists Act, when all dentists had to be registered, thereby excluding all charlatans and unqualified men. There is also a selection of dental chairs, tracing their development from the 16th century barber's chair to one used by Edward VII at Buckingham Palace.

The upper gallery has smaller items; dental instruments, equipment, decorative ceramics, prints and engravings.

BRITISH MUSEUM

GREAT RUSSELL STREET
LONDON WC1B 3DG

☎ TELEPHONE: 071-636 1555
OPEN: MONDAY - SATURDAY .... 10.00 - 5.00
              SUNDAY .... 2.30 - 6.00
ADMISSION: FREE
SHOP. REFRESHMENTS. TOILETS.

♿ DISABLED ACCESS RING 071-580 7384.

🕴 GUIDED TOURS. EDUCATIONAL PROGRAMMES.

The British Museum was founded on the library and collections of the physician, Sir Hans Sloane, which he bequeathed to the nation at his death in 1753, subject to a payment of £20,000. A home was eventually found in Bloomsbury in 1759 and to Sloane's original collections were added those of the Earls of Oxford, notably manuscripts and the library of the Cotton family. This became the first public secular museum in the world.

The British passion for travelling and collecting added many rich and important objects to the museum and to-day it spans the centuries from early civilisation to the present century. Many medical items can be found throughout the museum: the Babylonian clay model of a sheep's liver used for instruction in divination; an Egyptian papyri recommending magical cures for migraine, diseases affecting the bones, eyes and female organs and the body of 'Ginger' 3,400 years old; the mummies and canopic jars; the relief of the dying lioness, on the walls of the Palace of Assurbanipal, mortally wounded with her spinal cord severed whilst her mate vomits blood; a Greek statue of Aesculapius and Roman and Romano-British instruments and votive offerings.

The British Library, due to move to St. Pancreas very shortly, has the largest collection of manuscripts and medical texts.

BRITISH OPTICAL ASSOCIATION

FOUNDATION COLLECTION
c/o BRITISH COLLEGE OF OPTOMETRISTS
10 KNARESBOROUGH PLACE
LONDON SW5 0TG

ⓓ TELEPHONE: 071-373 7765
OPEN: MONDAY - FRIDAY ....10.00 - 4.00
             BY APPOINTMENT ONLY
ADMISSION: FREE

This fascinating collection of spectacles and optical aids dates from the Middle ages to the present day. Some examples of 16th and 17th century spectacles and their cases can be compared with later Chinese and Japanese varieties. The frames vary in material from brass, whalebone, tortoiseshell, balsa wood and iron, to silver and gilt. The spectacle cases show the ingenuity of the craftsmen and are often elaborately designed and decorated.

The 18th century and Regency period produced quizzers and spyglasses, often cunningly concealed in the top of a walking stick or in a fan. From 1820-1870 there are opera glasses, jealousy glasses, lorgnettes and semi-lorgnettes. A pair of 1920 surgeon's operating spectacles had long straight sides which allowed free movement up and down.

There is a collection of china figurines, bronze and wooden figures, sculptures and paintings all featuring spectacle wearers.

CHELSEA PHYSIC GARDEN

66 ROYAL HOSPITAL ROAD
LONDON SW3 4HS

ⓓ TELEPHONE: 071-352 5646
OPEN: WEDNESDAY & SUNDAY ....2.00 - 5.00
             MID MARCH - MID OCTOBER
             TUESDAY - FRIDAY ....CHELSEA SHOW WEEK
ADMISSION: CHARGE
SHOP. PLANTS FOR SALE. REFRESHMENTS. TOILETS.
♿ DISABLED ACCESS.

Founded in 1673 by the Society of Apothecaries, Chelsea Physic Garden is one of the oldest in Europe. In 1722 Sir Hans Sloane, having purchased the Manor of Chelsea, secured the future of the garden and presented it to the Society; his statue stands in the Garden. In 1732 cotton seed was sent to Georgia to help establish the industry there.

The 3.5 acres contain the oldest rock garden in Europe (1772), glasshouses, botanical order beds and an historical walk showing the variety of plant species introduced to Britain by a succession of famous curators. Amongst the trees is the largest outdoor olive tree in Britain which still produces fruit and a willow tree of the type depicted on 'Chinese Willow Pattern' plates.

The Garden still grows many medicinal plants including: artemesia for chloroquine-resistant cerebral malaria; the Madagascar periwinkle as the source of the cytoxic drugs vincristine and vinblastine; meadow saffron for gout; the woolly foxglove whose cardiac glycoside is digoxin; the mandrake whose root contains hyoscine; a tea-leafed willow whose active principle salicin is converted in the body into salicylic acid and the castor oil plant whose seed contains ricin currently being researched for use in the treatment of cancer.

The Garden is busy growing research material for medicine, monitoring the effect of the atmosphere on plants, particularly lichen, and exchanging plants and seeds with other botanical gardens throughout the world, but it still provides an oasis of quiet in the centre of a large city.

A library of herbals is available to view by appointment.

FLORENCE NIGHTINGALE MUSEUM

2 LAMBETH PALACE ROAD
LONDON SE1 7EW

℡ TELEPHONE: 071-620 0374
OPEN: TUESDAY - SUNDAY.................................10.00 - 4.00
              & B.H. MONDAYS
ADMISSION: CHARGE
SHOP. TOILETS.

♿ DISABLED ACCESS.

Florence Nightingale has gone down in history as the 'Lady with the Lamp', the nurse who walked among the wounded in the Crimean War in 1855. Her lamp and a ward at Scutari are shown in this excellent museum devoted to the life of this remarkable woman. An audio-visual programme shows the difficulties she encountered when it was unfashionable to train as a nurse, her experiences in the Crimea which led her to found the first school of nursing at St. Thomas's in 1860 and her campaigns to raise the standards of care and efficiency in hospitals and Army barracks, and amongst the poor.

Many of her personal letters and possessions, photographs, clothing and furniture are on display, including her room at South Street where she died in 1910 aged 90.

FREUD MUSEUM

20 MARESFIELD GARDENS
LONDON NW3 5SX

☎ TELEPHONE: 071-435 2002 / 5157
OPEN: WEDNESDAY - SUNDAY..............................12.00 - 5.00
ADMISSION: CHARGE
SHOP.

♿ DISABLED ACCESS TO GROUND FLOOR (INC. STUDY).

👫 PRE-BOOKED TOURS AT OTHER TIMES BY ARRANGEMENT.

In 1938, Sigmund Freud left his home in Vienna as a refugee to spend the last year of his life in exile in England. His unique and fascinating collection of Egyptian, Greek, Roman and Oriental antiquities came with him as did his famous couch and desk and many of his books. The rooms at Maresfield Gardens were his laboratory, the site of his discoveries about the human psyche, and they offer insights into the sources and nature of his achievements as the founder of psychoanalysis. His daughter, Anna, lived and worked here until her death in 1982 and a display upstairs shows the life and work of both father and daughter, including some rare 'home movies' taken of them both in the garden with friends and a favourite dog.

HAHNEMANN HOUSE TRUSTEES

2 POWIS PLACE
LONDON WC1N 3HT

☾ TELEPHONE: 071-837 9469
OPEN: BY APPOINTMENT ONLY TO THE ADMINISTRATOR.

The hospital first opened its doors at 32 Golden Square in 1849 after Dr. Frederick Quinn had introduced homeopathy to England. Quinn was physician to King Leopold of the Belgians, Queen Victoria'a uncle, and while travelling with him first learnt of homeopathy in Italy, later studying with Hahnemann in Paris. Back in England and moving in the highest social circles he brought respectability to treating 'like with like'.

In 1859 the Hospital moved to Great Ormond Street. The Hahnemann House Trustees, in an adjacent building, have relics belonging to Hahnemann including some minute bottles from his pocket medicine case which he used daily from 1835-43 and his cap and smoking hat. There are also some of the very small medicine tubes with their original contents, a globule chest and the mother tincture of arnica.

The Hahnemann House Trustees have much archive material and an exceptional reference library of homeopathic medicine with Kent's Repertory, Phatak's Materia Medica, Hahnemann's Chronic Diseases and Clarke's Materia Medica of 1900.

HMS BELFAST

MORGANS LANE
TOOLEY STREET
LONDON SE1 2JH

☾ TELEPHONE: 071-407 6434
OPEN: MONDAY - SUNDAY .... 10.00 - 5.50
MID-MARCH - END OCTOBER
.... 10.00 - 4.30
1ST NOVEMBER - MID-MARCH
ADMISSION: CHARGE
SHOP. REFRESHMENTS. TOILETS.

 ♿ DISABLED ACCESS TO UPPER DECK ONLY.

Lying in the Pool of London between Tower and London Bridges, HMS Belfast at 11,000 tons was in 1939 the largest cruiser ever built for the Royal Navy and is the last surviving warship of World War 2. During the war she fired the first shots in the Battle of North Cape in which the German battleship Scharnhorst was sunk. In 1944 she led the bombardment off the coast of Normandy.

HMS Belfast is now a floating museum and the entire ship is open to the public, from the gun turrets to the mess decks, bakery, machine shop, chapel, dental surgery and doctor's surgery, operating theatre and sick bay. In the theatre an operation is being carried out whilst the surgery shows some drug dispensing apparatus.

HUNTERIAN MUSEUM

ROYAL COLLEGE OF SURGEONS
LINCOLN'S INN FIELDS
LONDON WC2A 3PN

☎ TELEPHONE: 071-405 3474 EXT. 3011
    OPEN: MONDAY - FRIDAY ....10.00 - 5.00
               BY APPLICATION TO THE CURATOR ONLY
    ADMISSION: FREE

♿ DISABLED ACCESS.

The Company of Surgeons was established in 1745 after 200 years of uneasy alliance with the Barber-Surgeons. In 1800 the Company was granted a Royal Charter and became the Royal College of Surgeons in London and moved to a house in Lincoln's Inn Fields. It became the Royal College of Surgeons of England in 1843.

John Hunter, whose unique collection is at the College, was born in 1728 at Long Calderwood, East Kilbride. He was the youngest of 10 children and at the age of 20 he followed his elder brother, William, to London. William, a Surgeon Accoucheur at the Middlesex Hospital, ran his own Anatomy School. John joined him as his assistant, training at the same time under the surgeons Percival Pott and William

Cheselden, and qualified in medicine by 1755. He served in the Army for 3 years and on his return set up his own Anatomy School and practised surgery at St. George's Hospital.

John Hunter is rightly called 'the Father of Scientific Surgery' and his collection bears witness to his maxim: 'But why think, why not try the Experiment?'. It is his great unwritten book. His specimens have been arranged in three main groups:

1. Structures concerned in the preservation of the individual - how the body adapts to change
2. Structures concerned with the preservation of the race
3. Pathological conditions.

At his death in 1793 the museum contained 13,687 specimens which he wished to be offered to the British Government. Being short of funds it was not until 1799 that it was acquired and custody offered to the College of Surgeons.

In May 1941 the College received several direct hits during a bombing raid. Much was destroyed of the then 60,000 specimens including two fifths of Hunter's original collection.

Today the museum has re-assembled his unique collection according to his original concepts, and also includes some of his own instruments and other items of medical historical interest.

KEATS HOUSE

KEATS GROVE
HAMPSTEAD
LONDON NW3 2RR

☎ TELEPHONE: 081-435 2062
OPEN: MONDAY - FRIDAY ....2.00 - 6.00
        SATURDAY............................... 10.00 - 1.00 & 2.00 - 5.00
        SUNDAY & B.H. ....2.00 - 5.00
        APRIL - OCTOBER
        MONDAY - FRIDAY ....1.00 - 5.00
        SATURDAY & SUNDAY .... AS SUMMER
        NOVEMBER - MARCH
ADMISSION: FREE
SHOP.

  ♿ NO DISABLED ACCESS.

  👫 GUIDED TOURS FOR PARTIES.

John Keats passed the examination for the licence of the Worshipful Society of Apothecaries on July 25th 1816, having spent four years apprenticed to Thomas Hammond of Edmonton and 'walking the wards' at Guy's Hospital. Although qualified to practice medicine, he never did so and passed the rest of his short life as a poet, dying of tuberculosis at the age of 25 in Rome.

The two lovely Regency semi-detached cottages, built in 1815-16, now made into one house, are where Keats spent his most creative years following the death of his brother Tom in 1818. It was here also that he fell in love with Fanny Brawne. The house contains relics, books, manuscripts, portraits and letters and has been preserved very much as a home.

LONDON CHEST HOSPITAL

> BONNER ROAD
> LONDON E2 9JX

  ☎ TELEPHONE: 081-980 2215
      OPEN: BY APPOINTMENT ONLY FOR SERIOUS
               RESEARCHERS. APPLY TO DR. S.J. STEEL,
               HONORARY ARCHIVIST.

The hospital came to the East End in 1851 from its previous home in Liverpool Street and was called the City of London Hospital for Diseases of the Lungs, specialising in diseases of the heart and lungs, in particular tubercular cases. Sir Joseph Paxton promised to design a crystal sanatorium, but in the end this proved too expensive to build. When fresh-air was the chosen cure, galleries were added to the wards, some of which still remain.

The instruments on display include a MacKenzie and Lewis E.C.G. polygraph of 1920, infusion apparatus, a pulse recorder of 1900, aspiration sets, Lister's carbolic spray, bronchoscopes for use with local anaesthetic, Lillingston

Pearson pneumothorax apparatus of the early 1900's, a Stott machine and a Maxwell box.

The archive material includes doctor's notes from 1902, matron's diary and the minutes of the Governor's meetings.

MUSEUM OF LONDON

LONDON WALL
LONDON EC2Y 5HN

☎ TELEPHONE: 071-600 3699
OPEN: TUESDAY - SATURDAY .... 10.00 - 6.00
SUNDAY .... 12.00 - 6.00
OPEN B.H. MONDAYS
ADMISSION: CHARGE
SHOP. REFRESHMENTS. TOILETS.
♿ DISABLED ACCESS.

In the Barbican complex the Museum of London chronicles the history of the City from the early settlers and the Roman invasion in 43 A.D. and the founding of Londinium, through the Dark Ages, Medieval years, Tudor, Stuart and Georgian times to the 19th and 20th centuries.

The medical practices of London physicians, barber-surgeons, apothecaries and hospitals are to be found in these periods, beginning with a Book of Regulations of 1588 from the Royal College of Physicians and an order sheet on street cleaning and hygiene to try and control epidemics. There is an example of cinchona bark used to treat malaria, silver pomanders, 17th century pewter and brass syringes, surgical instruments, spectacles and a bleeding bowl.

In the 18th century are examples of medicine bottles, Bills of Mortality (weekly returns of deaths from 109 parishes), a travelling tooth-brush, cupping set, small wood medicine chest and a prescription for Lady Rose in 1790. There is a display on the work of Dr. Barnardo who in 1867, founded homes for destitute and neglected children and a 19th century reconstructed pharmacy.

MUSEUM OF THE ORDER OF ST. JOHN

ST. JOHN'S GATE
ST. JOHN'S LANE
CLERKENWELL
LONDON EC1M 4DA

☎ TELEPHONE: 071-253 6644
OPEN: MONDAY - FRIDAY ....10.00 - 5.00
SATURDAY...10.00 - 4.00
ADMISSION: FREE, DONATION REQUESTED
SHOP. TOILETS.

& DISABLED ACCESS.

The Tudor gatehouse of the Priory of the Knights Hospitaller traces the history of the Order from their early work in Jerusalem, when a hospital was established to look after the sick pilgrims and wounded during the Crusades, to the Ophthalmic Hospital they staff to-day. The Order was expelled from the Middle East in 1291 and moved to Cyprus, Rhodes and Malta. To-day their headquarters is in Rome. The museum has a beautifully illustrated Order of Service, the Rhodes Missal, some rare Rhodes armour and highly decorated drug jars.

After the Reformation the Order was dissolved in England until 1877 when it was re-formed as the St. John Ambulance Association to continue the Hospitaller tradition of looking after the sick by providing first-aid training. In 1888 the St. John Ambulance Brigade gave a voluntary first aid service for the public. Their first aid equipment, uniforms and medals are on display. A small room is devoted to the work of the Ophthalmic Hospital in Jerusalem, founded in 1882, which treats patients regardless of race, colour or creed.

The Order has a number of medieval chapels and almshouses around the country, notable Coningsby Hospital, Hereford which has a small museum, and St. John's Jerusalem Garden and Chapel at Sutton-at-Hone, Dartford.

MUSEUM OF THE ROYAL PHARMACEUTICAL SOCIETY OF GREAT BRITAIN

1 LAMBETH HIGH STREET
LONDON SW1 7JN

☎ TELEPHONE: 071-735 9141
OPEN: MONDAY - FRIDAY
BY APPOINTMENT ONLY FOR SERIOUS
RESEARCHERS ON APPLICATION TO THE
MUSEUM CURATOR

Founded in 1841 and granted a Royal charter in 1843 the Royal Pharmaceutical Society is the registration and professional body for pharmacists in all aspects of practice. In 1892 the Daniel Hanbury (1825-75) bequest formed the basis of a remarkable library and a fascinating collection of old herbals, pill making equipment, pharmaceutical ceramics, dispensing equipment, prints and photographs.

NATIONAL ARMY MUSEUM

ROYAL HOSPITAL ROAD
CHELSEA
LONDON SW3

☎ TELEPHONE: 071-730 0717
OPEN: MONDAY - SUNDAY .... 10.00 - 5.30
ADMISSION: FREE
SHOP. REFRESHMENTS. TOILETS.
♿ DISABLED ACCESS.
👥 EDUCATIONAL SERVICES. CONFERENCE FACILITIES.

This museum, devoted to the story of the British soldier in peace and war from Tudor times to the present day, has a fascinating display of models, reconstructions, personal relics, medals, paintings, uniforms, weapons, silver and vehicles.

Amongst the vehicles is a Ford jeep used for casualty evacuation with a casualty on a stretcher, a stretcher used for the D-day landings and the uniform of a sergeant in the RAMC in 1918 and a FANY, a nurse in the First Aid

Nursing Yeomanry. There is also a lamp used by Florence Nightingale in Scutari.

PETER PAN GALLERY

55 GREAT ORMOND STREET
LONDON WC1

✆ TELEPHONE: 071-405 9200 EXT. 5920
OPEN: MONDAY - FRIDAY .... BY APPOINTMENT
ADMISSION: FREE
♿ NO DISABLED ACCESS

The Hospital for Sick Children opened in February 1852 largely as the inspiration of Dr Charles West. This story is told by photographs, memorabilia and ephemera in this small but fascinating museum. Amongst West's supporters were such eminent men as Charles Dickens, one of whose speeches can be seen, and Lord Shaftsbury. Newspaper articles follow the progress of the hospital. There is also on display a manuscript of Sir James Barrie's speech of 1930 asking for funds. He gave the hospital a lasting memorial and money-raiser by assigning to them the copyright and performing rights of the story of "Peter Pan" (the boy who never grew up). The "Bombing Book" is a facsimile of the signatures of presidents, prime minister, actors and actresses who campaigned for the rebuilding of the hospital after bomb damage in the Second World War. Some surgical apparatus of 1875, a doctor's wartime case, lists of nurse's lectures and rules and regulations for the patients are on display, together with clothes worn by the children in 1893 and a small wheel-chair. The archive material is available on request.

RAGGED SCHOOL MUSEUM

46-50 COPPERFIELD ROAD
BOW
LONDON E3 4RR

✆ TELEPHONE: 081-980 6405

OPEN: WEDNESDAY & THURSDAY .... 10.00 - 5.00
               1ST SUNDAY OF THE MONTH
ADMISSION: FREE. DONATIONS APPRECIATED
SHOP. REFRESHMENTS. TOILETS.

  NO DISABLED ACCESS.

  EDUCATION PROGRAMME.

The two warehouses, built in 1872 next to the Regent's Canal, were rented 5 years later by Dr. Barnardo as Free Ragged Day and Sunday Schools for children from the poorest families in the district. By 1879 they were the largest Ragged Day School in London. Unlike the London Board Schools which charged a penny or more a week, the Ragged School also gave free breakfast and dinner in the winter. Evening classes were held for factory girls and from 1884 a Working Lads' Institute. The schools were closed in 1908 and the Sunday School in 1916 when the lease ran out. For the next 60 years the buildings were mostly used by Jewish clothing manufacturers.

The museum concentrates on the experiences of the children who attended Dr. Barnardo's school. There is a reconstructed Victorian class-room where to-day's children can participate in a Victorian school lesson. The upper floor examines the possibilities of work for the children once they left the Ragged School either in service, a sewing shop, a laundry for girls, as a City messenger or part of the wood chopping brigade for the boys.

There is an area of temporary exhibitions and a display of the East End during the second World War.

ROYAL COLLEGE OF OBSTETRICIANS & GYNAECOLOGISTS

27 SUSSEX PLACE
REGENT'S PARK
LONDON NW1 4RG

TELEPHONE: 071-262 5425 EXT. 213
OPEN: MONDAY - FRIDAY .... 10.00 - 5.00
               FOR SERIOUS RESEARCHERS ONLY ON
               APPLICATION TO THE LIBRARIAN

It was opposition from the other Royal Colleges that delayed the founding of the Royal College of Obstetricians and Gynaecologists until 25th September 1929, first as a company, then receiving a Royal charter in 1938 and finally moving to Regent's Park in July 1960.

The comprehensive collection of obstetric and gynaecological instruments has on show the original Chamberlen forceps. The Chamberlens were a Huguenot family who fled to England in 1569. They settled in London and two brothers became members of the Barber Surgeons Company where they tried unsuccessfully to form a guild of midwives. Being innovators and opportunists it was Peter the Elder (d1631) who probably devised the original forceps which had, uniquely, an articulation or locking device using tape passed through a hole in each blade and wound round the handle. Great secrecy surrounded this invention until the early 18th century when the true details 'leaked' out. They were lost for 150 years until discovered in 1813 under a trap door in an attic at Woodham Mortimer Hall, the home of Dr. Peter.

Other instruments include those by Smellie, Chapman, Hamilton, Davies, J.Y. Simpson, Clover and Kielland.

ROYAL HOSPITAL

ROYAL HOSPITAL ROAD
CHELSEA
LONDON SW3 4SL

☎ TELEPHONE: 071-730 0161
OPEN: MONDAY - FRIDAY .... 10.00 - 12.00 & 2.00 - 6.00
ADMISSION: FREE
SHOP. TOILETS.

♿ DISABLED ACCESS.

🕴 GROUPS BY ARRANGEMENT.

The imposing and magnificent building by Sir Christopher Wren opened in 1682 as a retreat for veteran soldiers of the regular army who had become unfit for duty, either after 20 years' service or as a result of wounds. To-day the In-Pensioners number about 400, are not normally less than 65 years of age, are boarded, lodged and clothed and receive medical care and a small weekly allowance.

Both the Great Hall and Chapel are open to the public. There is a small museum entered through the Wellington Hall with paintings of the Battle of Waterloo. The long gallery has prints, photographs, arms, uniforms and other items associated with the hospital including a plan of the burial ground where William Cheselden the 18th century surgeon and lithotomist is buried.

SPRINGFIELD HOSPITAL MUSEUM

61 GLENBURNIE ROAD
LONDON SW17 7DJ

☎ TELEPHONE: 081-672 9911 EXT. 42463
OPEN: BY APPOINTMENT ONLY

This psychiatric hospital has a fascinating archive collection of case notes, admission sheets, ward report books, personal details of diagnosis, treatment and discharge of the 1850's, committee books and agendas from 1841-1950. The small museum room has photographs of the original founders of the then 'Surrey County Lunatic Asylum' in 1840 who included William Cubitt, younger brother of Thomas the speculator and builder who developed the Duke of Bedford's estate in Bloomsbury and Pimlico.

Items on display are a strong shirt, 1920; scissors with a leather scabbard; removable bath taps; apothecary's scales; tracheotomy set (because choking on food was quite common); a notebook recording commissioners informal interviews with patients, 1910-1946; and an engineer's log book, 1899.

THE NATURAL HISTORY MUSEUM

CROMWELL ROAD
LONDON SW7 5BD

☎ TELEPHONE: 071-938 9123

```
OPEN:    MONDAY - SATURDAY ............................... 10.00 - 17.50
         SUNDAY ....................................................... 11.00 - 17.50
ADMISSION: CHARGE
SHOP. REFRESHMENTS. TOILETS. SPECIAL EVENTS.
LECTURES.
```
  ♿   DISABLED ACCESS.

This magnificent building designed by Alfred Waterhouse (1873-80) is the home of the original natural history collection of Sir Hans Sloane, which was part of the British Museum.

The galleries are divided into Life Galleries and Earth Galleries. The former include the dinosaurs, fish and reptiles, ecology, minerals, plants, mammals, and human biology. This hall shows how the body works with large scale models, diagrams, and audio-visual displays. Man's place in evolution on the first floor examines how we are related to the fossil humans that have already been discovered.

The Earth Galleries examine how resources from the Earth from fuels to precious metals are used in our daily lives, with exhibitions on earthquakes, Britain before man, fossils, rocks, geological surveys and minerals.

THE OLD OPERATING THEATRE MUSEUM & HERB GARRET

```
ST. THOMAS'S CHURCH
9A ST. THOMAS'S STREET
SOUTHWARK
LONDON SE1 9RT
```

☎ TELEPHONE: 071-955 4791 / 081-806 4325
```
    OPEN:    TUESDAY - SUNDAY ..................................... 10.00 - 4.00
    ADMISSION: CHARGE
    SHOP.
```
  ♿   NO DISABLED ACCESS, ACCESS DIFFICULT UP A SPIRAL STAIRWAY.

  🚶 GROUPS BY ARRANGEMENT.

The Church was the Hospital Chapel and the roof used as a herb garret by the hospital apothecary. In 1821 it was decided that the female patients needed their own operating theatre, as operating on the ward was noisy and distressing for other patients. Being on the same level as the Herb Garret and finding suitable space in the roof, an operating theatre was created and used until 1863 when the entire hospital re-located further up river to its present site.

To-day the operating theatre is complete with 'standings' for the students, original table, chairs, wash bowl and mop and leather bucket for washing the floor. To prevent any blood from seeping through the floor boards onto the heads of the congregation below, sawdust was packed between the boards and a box filled with sawdust kept under the operating table to catch any sudden excess of blood!

The herb garret has a collection of old instruments, fleams, cupping sets, pathology specimens, nursing equipment, plants used in medicine and a display on the history of the hospital and the influence of Florence Nightingale.

THE ROYAL LONDON HOSPITAL MUSEUM & ARCHIVES CENTRE

ST. AUGUSTINE WITH ST. PHILIP'S CHURCH
NEWARK STREET
LONDON E1 2AA

℡ TELEPHONE: 071-377 7000 EXT. 3364
OPEN: MONDAY - FRIDAY .... 10.00 - 4.30
ADMISSION: FREE, DONATION REQUESTED
SHOP.

& DISABLED ACCESS TO ALL MUSEUM.

👫 GROUPS AND GUIDED TOURS BY ARRANGEMENT.

Opened in 1989 in the basement of a fine 19th century early English style church, the museum provides a home for records of health care in Tower Hamlets, including the extensive series of archives of the Royal London Hospital, dating from its foundation in 1740.

A display of photographs, written material, ephemera and uniforms looks at the history of the London Hospital and the contribution of such medical pioneers as Sir Frederick Treves and Dr. Barnardo as well as Edith Cavell. Modern developments such as London's first Helicopter Emergency Service are the subject or temporary displays.

THE THOMAS CORAM FOUNDATION FOR CHILDREN

40 BRUNSWICK SQUARE
LONDON WC1N 1AZ

☏ TELEPHONE: 071-278 2424
OPEN: MONDAY - FRIDAY ....10.00 - 4.00
ADMISSION: CHARGE
SHOP. TOILETS.

 NO DISABLED ACCESS.

 ROOMS USED FOR MEETINGS, RING FIRST.

Thomas Coram was the originator of the first major institution to care for children in England. Born in 1668 he went to sea aged 11 years and spent most of his life either at sea or in shipbuilding. His travels to the 'New Colonies' made him appreciate the value of human life in building up a new country. Thus he was distressed to see on his visits to London so many young children abandoned in the gutters and left to die on the dung heaps.

Determined to provide a solution for the problem he gained enough support to successfully petition George II and so opened his Foundling Hospital in 1739 on the present Coram Fields. Richard Mead and William Hogarth were both patrons and Hogarth's splendid portrait of the founder still hangs at the top of the stairs. In 1926 the Governors decided to move the Hospital to the cleaner air of the country, first to Redhill then to Berkhamsted (closed 1953). The original hospital in London was demolished and a new headquarters built in 1937, since when the Hospital had changed emphasis to become an adoption agency, with a children's centre, day nursery and nursery school.

In the Court Room with its splendidly ornate ceiling are 8 small painted roundels of the principal London hospitals of the day and glass cases with tokens and trinkets left with children by their mothers. In the Picture Gallery are paintings, uniforms worn by the children and a number of objects associated with Handel (another supporter), including a fair copy of the Messiah and the keyboard of the original organ on which he played many times.

THE SIR ALEXANDER FLEMING LABORATORY MUSEUM

ST. MARY'S HOSPITAL
PRAED STREET
LONDON W2 1NY

☎ TELEPHONE: 071-725 6528
   OPEN: BY APPOINTMENT ONLY TO THE ARCHIVIST

♿ NO DISABLED ACCESS.

🚶 GROUPS BY ARRANGEMENT.

This new museum is hoping to open by Easter 1993. The Hospital and Medical School are reconstructing the small laboratory used by Sir Alexander Fleming in 1928 when he discovered penicillin. One exhibition will show his life and work and that of Chain and Florey, the other the impact of penicillin on medicine with its far reaching effects.

THE WELLCOME MUSEUM OF THE HISTORY OF MEDICINE

THE SCIENCE MUSEUM
EXHIBITION ROAD
LONDON SW7 2DD

☎ TELEPHONE: 071-938 8000
   OPEN: MONDAY - SATURDAY .... 10.00 - 6.00
                 SUNDAY .... 11.00 - 6.00
   ADMISSION: CHARGE
   SHOP. REFRESHMENTS. TOILETS.

♿ DISABLED ACCESS TO ALL FLOORS.

🚶 GROUPS BY ARRANGEMENT. PRE-BOOKED EDUCATIONAL PARTIES FREE.

The museum houses Britain's greatest collection of science and industry, with examples and illustrations of machines, apparatus and scientific discovery. From Stephenson's Rocket to the Apollo 10 spacecraft the diversity of the objects range through transport, food, chemicals, mechanical apparatus, power, optics, telecommunications, geophysics, photography and medicine.

The two floors of Medical History are due largely to the collecting zeal of Sir Henry Wellcome. During the last 40 years of his life (he died in 1936) he amassed a vast number of objects, books, letters and paintings, many of which have been on display at the Science Museum since 1982.

The 'Science of Art and Medicine' has a chronological display of medical items from the Egyptians, Greeks and Romans to 20th century laboratory medicine, the influences of conflict and exploration on medicine, and medicine in the third world.

The gallery on the 4th floor, 'Glimpses of Medical History' contains a series of reconstructions, dioramas and models from a Neolithic trepanning operation to a 1980 heart operation.

A large gallery is also devoted to veterinary medicine.

UNIVERSITY COLLEGE

UNIVERSITY OF LONDON
GOWER STREET
LONDON WC1E 6BT

☎ TELEPHONE: 071-387 7050
OPEN: MONDAY - FRIDAY ....10.00 - 5.00
ADMISSION: FREE
 NO DISABLED ACCESS.

The imposing Wilkins building in the University has a scattered collection of medical items relating to past Professors and lecturers of the University.

Instruments for the removal of bladder stones, belonging to Sir Henry Thompson, Professor of Clinical Surgery 1865-75; a display and photographs of William Squire, the 21 year old medical student who administered the first ether anaesthetic in 1846 for Robert Liston; a microscope used by Edmond Grant FRS, Professor of Comparative Anatomy and Zoology 1828-74; the first X-ray photograph used for clinical purposes in this country taken by Norman Collie in 1896, showing the broken needle in the thumb of the patient. A model of DNA commemorates Francis Crick who jointly won the Nobel Prize in 1962 for the discovery of DNA.

The most unusual exhibit is the clothed skeleton of the philosopher and founder of the College, Jeremy Bentham, which he bequeathed to the College.

WELLCOME CENTRE FOR MEDICAL SCIENCE & HISTORY

183 EUSTON ROAD
LONDON NW1 2BN

☎ TELEPHONE: 071-611 8727   INFORMATION LINE
OPEN: MONDAY - FRIDAY ....9.45 - 5.00
               EXHIBITION & INFORMATION CENTRE ONLY
               SATURDAY..9.45 - 12.30
ADMISSION: FREE
BOOK SHOP.
♿ DISABLED ACCESS.

The Wellcome Centre has undergone a complete change over the past year and now has a new permanent exhibition on modern medical science entitled Science for Life. The exhibition aims to show the different aspects of medical science and biomedical research and how their work is supported.

The Information Centre will provide background information on medical research, biomedical research policy, funding, management, organisation and manpower, together with non-technical summaries of current developments and career opportunities in research. There will be a programme of scientific meetings and seminars and access to the new Tropical Diseases Videodisc.

Two History of Medicine exhibitions are being developed in the building, one a general introduction to the subject entitled Medicine in Time which covers specific topics, such as Plagues and People, Hospitals, The Clinical Encounter, Pharmacopoeia and Science and Medicine. A series of changing exhibits on the fourth floor covers different aspects of medicine relating to the collections held at The Wellcome.

The Wellcome Institute for the History of Medicine has a programme of meetings, research seminars, symposiums and public lectures.

WESLEY'S HOUSE & MUSEUM

47 CITY ROAD
LONDON EC1Y 1AU

ⓓ TELEPHONE: 071-253 2262
OPEN: MONDAY - SATURDAY...............................10.00 - 4.00
ADMISSION: CHARGE
SHOP. TOILETS.
♿ NO DISABLED ACCESS TO HOUSE.

John Wesley, the Methodist leader, lived in this plain and simple Georgian house from 1779 to his death in 1791. It contains many of his personal items, letters, clothes, books, travelling case and pieces of furniture.

Wesley was very interested in medicine and wrote a book 'Primitive Physick, or, an Easy and Natural Method of Curing most Disease' in which he attempted to provide a plain and easy way of curing most diseases. He regarded prayer as an addition to rather than a substitute for theriacs and medicines. In 1760 he published a book on 'Electricity made Plain and Useful' having already purchased a machine and successfully cured several patients. That electrotherapy machine is in his house in City Road.

The Museum, under the Chapel, depicts the lives of both John and Charles, the spread of Methodism and its influence in the world.

Norfolk

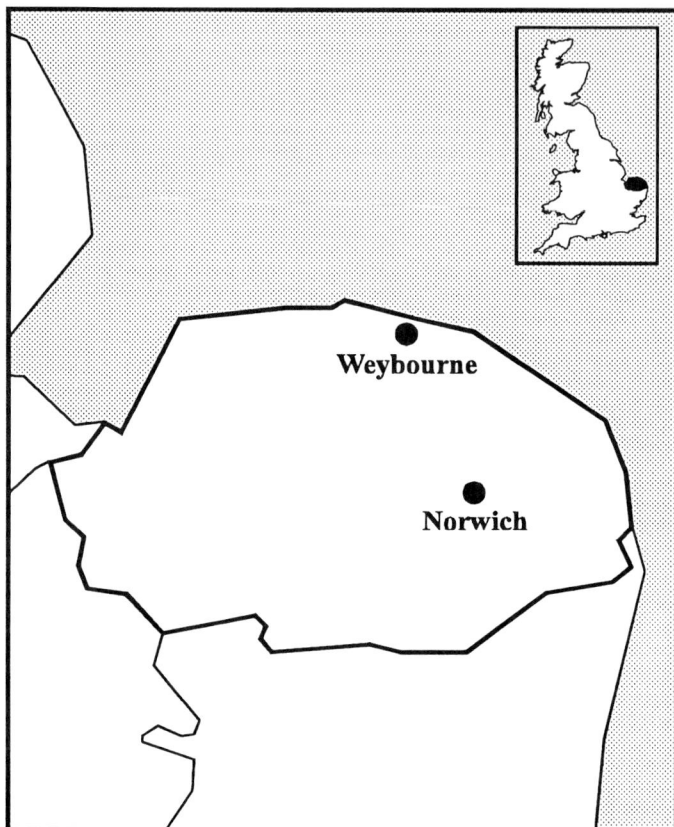

BRIDEWELL MUSEUM OF NORWICH TRADES & INDUSTRIES

BRIDEWELL ALLEY
ST. ANDREW'S STREET
NORWICH
NORFOLK NR2 1AQ

TELEPHONE: 0603-667 228
OPEN: MONDAY - SATURDAY .... 10.00 - 5.00
ADMISSION: CHARGE
SHOP. TOILETS.

NO DISABLED ACCESS.

In a building that was once a prison, tobacco factory, leather warehouse and boot and shoe factory, the museum was first established in 1925. Devoted to goods and services made in, or used by the people of Norwich, the museum displays items from the grain trade, iron founding and engineering, textile industry, shoemaking, brewing, printing and building. The pharmacy, early 20th century, has a mahogany drug run with the abbreviated Latin names for their contents, glass jars and bottles, eye-testing charts with symbols for the illiterate, baby weighing scales and a list of '50 DONT'S for the use of Chemists, their Assistants and Apprentices'. One of them reads, "Don't make fun of the customers who ask for 'hikey pikey' etc., they know what they want, and are ready to pay for it." Hikey pikey meant Hiera Picra, a compound of aloes and canella bark used as both a laxative and a tonic.

THE MUCKLEBURGH COLLECTION

WEYBOURNE MILITARY CAMP
WEYBOURNE
NORFOLK NR25 7EG

☎ TELEPHONE: 026-370 210/608
    OPEN: MONDAY - SUNDAY ....10.00 - 5.00
              MID-MARCH - NOVEMBER 1ST
    ADMISSION: CHARGE
    SHOP. REFRESHMENTS. TOILETS. SPECIAL EVENT DAYS.
    WORKING DISPLAYS OF TANKS ON BANK HOLIDAYS.

♿ DISABLED ACCESS.

🚶 PRE-BOOK EVENING PARTIES.

The largest private military collection in the United Kingdom of heavy armour, artefacts and models. This unique museum represents 'living military history', with exhibits from working WW2 tanks to Iraqi A.A. guns captured in Kuwait. There is a complete Austin K2 Ambulance, with its total kit as used in WW2, including splints, bandages etc. and a Dodge USA Ambulance as used in Vietnam complete with stretchers and first aid kit. RAMC badges and uniforms are on display as is an exhibition of the Suffolk and Norfolk Yeomanry regiment.

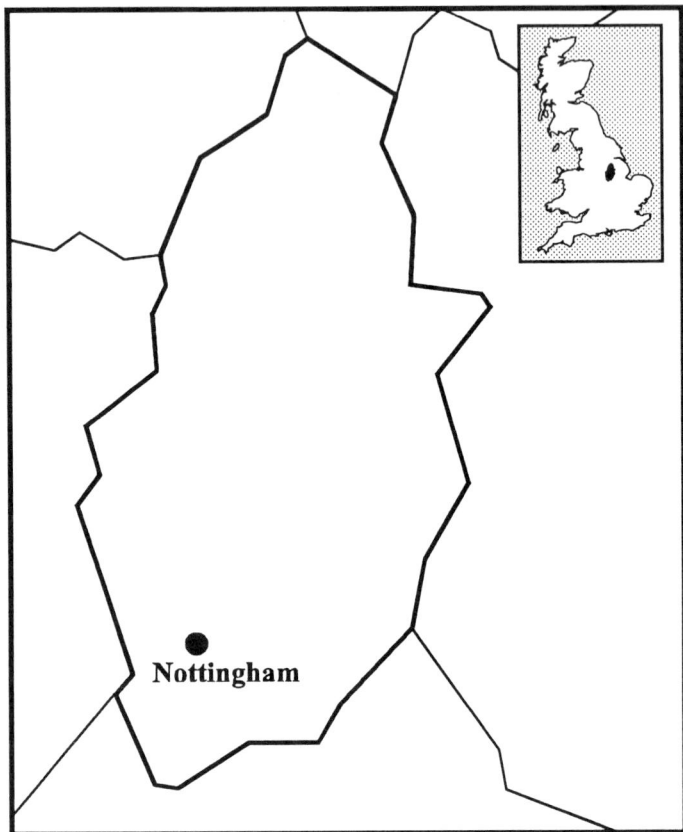

BREWHOUSE YARD MUSEUM

CASTLE BOULEVARD
NOTTINGHAM NG7 1FB

TELEPHONE: 0602-483 504
OPEN: MONDAY - SUNDAY .... 10.00 - 5.00
ADMISSION: FREE
SHOP & REFRESHMENTS AT CASTLE. TOILETS.

DISABLED ACCESS TO GROUND FLOOR ONLY.

Aspects of daily life in Nottingham are shown in these five 17th century houses opened in 1977 and 1978. Period rooms, shops, rock-cut caves, models and display cases are used to give glimpses into Nottingham's past with all the items displayed either made or used in the local area. The caves or rock-cellars hewn into the Castle rock behind the houses have been used for ale cellarage, workshops, wash houses and more recently W.W.2 air raid shelters. Changes in domestic life are shown through a series of period rooms and the newly opened shopping street displays a range of sales stock from 1919 - 1939. The walk-in chemist's shop contains material from 1880-1920 from various local chemists including a drug-run, bottles, jars, pots of ointments, pill making equipment, instructions on how to apply bandages and a Nelson inhaler. A Doctor's surgery with dispensing area, c.1930, can also be seen. The museum hopes to hold the historic material from Mapperley Mental Hospital but, as it is unlikely to be on display immediately, would be available only by prior appointment.

Oxfordshire

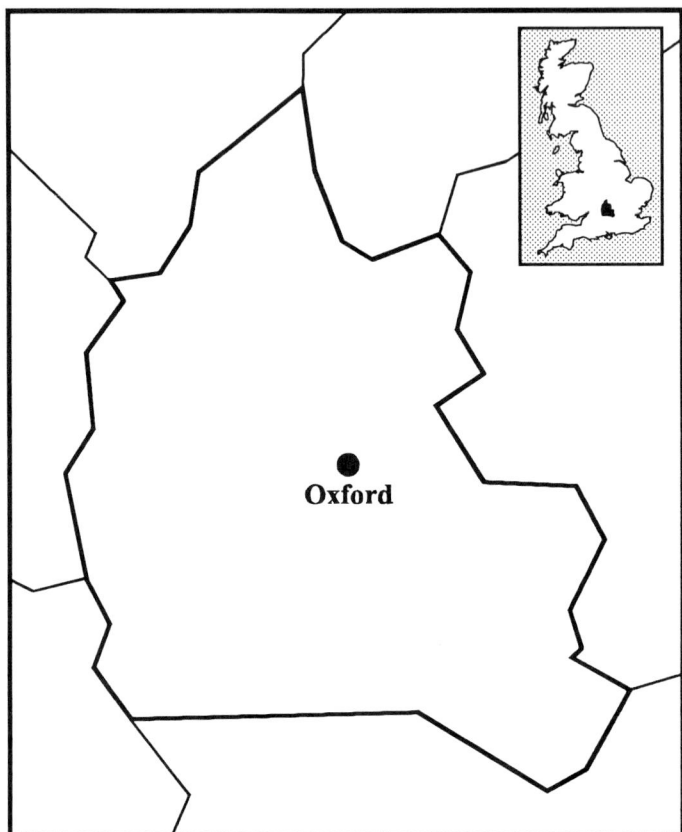

BOTANIC GARDEN

ROSE LANE
OXFORD
OXFORDSHIRE OXI 4AX

☎ TELEPHONE: 0865-276 920
OPEN: MONDAY - SUNDAY ....9.00 - 5.00
CLOSES: IN WINTER..4.30
GREENHOUSES..2.00 - 4.00
ADMISSION: FREE EXCEPT JULY & AUGUST

♿ DISABLED ACCESS ON GRAVEL PATHS.

Oxford's Botanic Garden is the third oldest in the world after Pisa and Leiden. In 1621 Henry Danvers gave £5,000 to the University to set up a Physic Garden for the use of the University and the people. The land chosen had been a Jewish cemetery until 1290, lying outside the city wall. The first operation was to raise the level of the land above the river Cherwell floodwater. To this end, 4,000 loads of 'muckle and donge' were spread, then a 14 foot wall was built round the 2.5 acre site. The first Superintendent was Jacob Bobart, succeeded by his son Bobart the Younger. It was due to them that the London Plane tree was introduced into England.

From the outset the purpose of the Garden was to support the study of medicine. To-day the Garden has culinary, dye and medicinal herbs, plants that are grown for their fibres, those used in the perfumery trade and examples of some of the most important food crop plants in the world. The Historical Rose display, wall plants, trees, rock garden and bog garden make this a unique and diverse collection of plants.

MUSEUM OF THE HISTORY OF SCIENCE

OLD ASHMOLEAN BUILDING
BROAD STREET
OXFORD
OXFORDSHIRE OX1 3AZ

☏ TELEPHONE: 0865-277 280
OPEN: MONDAY - FRIDAY .... 10.30 - 1.00 & 2.30 - 4.00
ADMISSION: FREE

♿ DISABLED ACCESS DIFFICULT - STEPS TO MUSEUM ENTRANCE.

The Old Ashmolean Building was built between 1679 and 1683, possibly by Thomas Wood, and is one of the finest 17th century buildings in the City. Occupied since 1935 by the Museum of the History of Science it has an unparalleled collection of early astronomical and mathematical instruments and an almost complete series of early microscopes (an 1880 copy of Leunhoek's microscope and a 1920 silver plated version) and other optical instruments. Clocks and watches, air-pumps, frictional electrical machines and other instruments of physics and early chemical apparatus, including some chemical glassware from the Daubeny Laboratory. At present the basement houses the medical collection which includes instruments (fleams, trepanning sets, scarifiers), some wet specimens, a wax model used at Christ Church, an ivory mannequin, a small bronze 'muscle man', an early artificial elbow joint, dental instruments, patent medicines, homeopathic remedies, medical amulets and Lister's carbolic spray. There are some early X-ray tubes, an induction machine used by Capt. Churchill when a student and later in the Boer War. The excellent library is open to research students on application to the Librarian.

A public space in the nearby John Radcliffe Hospital has on show the Macintosh collection of early anaesthetic equipment, and also an example of the Haldane apparatus.

OXFORD UNIVERSITY MUSEUM

PARKS ROAD
OXFORD
OXFORDSHIRE

☎ TELEPHONE; 0865-272 950
OPEN: MONDAY - SATURDAY .... 10.00 - 5.00
ADMISSION: FREE
SHOP. TOILETS.

♿ DISABLED ACCESS TO GROUND FLOOR.

Built in 1855/60 in the Neo-Gothic style, popular with the Pre-Raphaelite philosophy of the time, the museum surrounds a large courtyard with a massive roof supported by cast-iron pillars. The upper and lower arcades are themselves supported by columns of polished stone each of a different British rock whose capitals are beautifully carved with individual natural forms. Various statues in the courtyard commemorate men of science, including Aristotle,

Hippocrates, Harvey, Sydenham, John Hunter, Priestley, Davy and Charles Darwin.

The museum is the home of a large natural history collection, originally part of Elias Ashmole's museum, with some early specimens from the Tradescant family, 17th century gardeners and collectors, whose specimens formed the nucleus of the Ashmolean Museum. Also transferred from the Ashmolean were the collections of the explorer William Burchell, William Buckland the geologist, and osteological and physiological material from the Christ Church Museum, which had been assembled for medical teaching by Sir Henry Acland. Also a vast collection of insects and crustaceans donated in 1849 by the Rev. Hope.

There is an exhibition of plants in medicine.

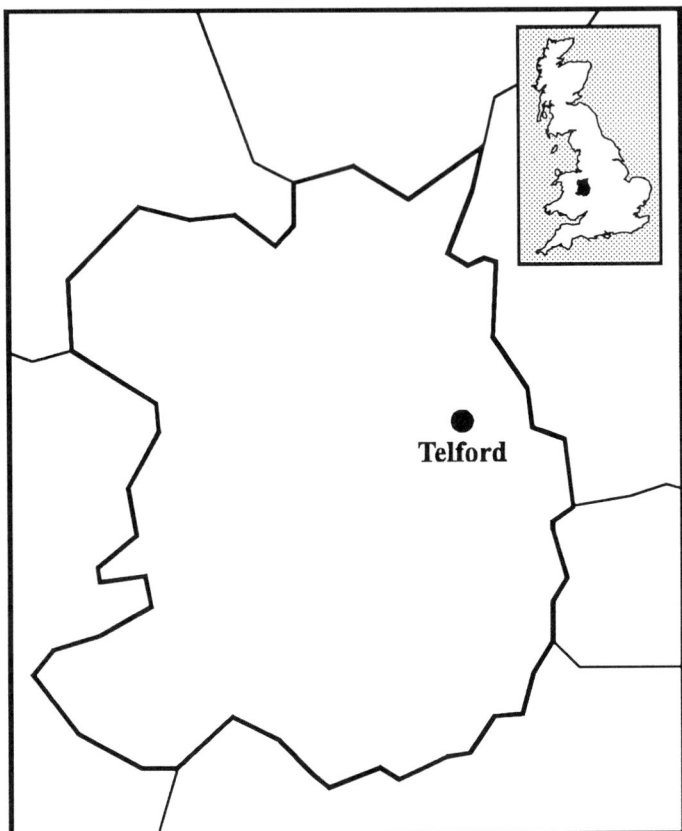

THE IRONBRIDGE GORGE MUSEUM

IRONBRIDGE
TELFORD
SHROPSHIRE TF8 7AW

TELEPHONE: 0952-433 522 (0952-432 166 W/E)
OPEN: MONDAY - SUNDAY .... 10.00 - 5.00
            EXCEPT JUNE, JULY, AUGUST
CLOSES: 6.00
            SMALLER SITES CLOSED IN WINTER
ADMISSION: CHARGE. PASSPORT TICKET FOR ADMISSION
TO ALL MUSEUM SITES AT ANY TIME IN THE FUTURE.

SHOPS. REFRESHMENTS. TOILETS.
PARK AND RIDE BUS SERVICE BETWEEN MUSEUM SITES.
FREE PARKING AT MOST MUSEUMS.

Spread over nearly 6 square miles, 6 Museums, a visitor centre, Quaker iron-master's house, Tar Tunnel and the famous Iron Bridge and Tollhouse combine to give an insight into the birth of the Industrial Revolution. Here were made the first iron rails, the first iron wheels, iron boat, cast-iron bridge and even the first high pressure steam locomotive. Here too, fine china developed at Coalport, stunning tiles at Jackfield and revolutionary transport systems.

At **BLISTS HILL OPEN AIR MUSEUM**, a town on a 50 acre site, the sometimes original, sometimes reconstructed buildings take the visitor back to life at the turn of the century. It has a butcher, baker and candlestick maker, a pub and foundry, carpenter's shop, coal mine and sweet shop. A bank to change money into pennies and farthings to spend in the shops. The Chemist's shop has a wide range of herbs and spices for sale to-day, but a 100 years ago sold patent medicines, toiletries, quack's cures, and prepared prescriptions. Also an opticians corner, with a sight testing chart of pictures for the illiterate, and assorted spectacles together with a small dental surgery, for the monthly visiting dentist ensured the townspeople were well looked after. The local Doctor had his surgery in his own home, and the small sparse waiting room led to his consulting room in the 'back room', enabling him to examine patients and possibly perform some minor operations.

THE JACKFIELD TILE MUSEUM has examples of tiles as pictorial panels which were a popular decoration for shops and hospitals. The Wendy House panel is from the children's ward of the King Edward VII Memorial Hospital, Ealing in 1930.

Somerset

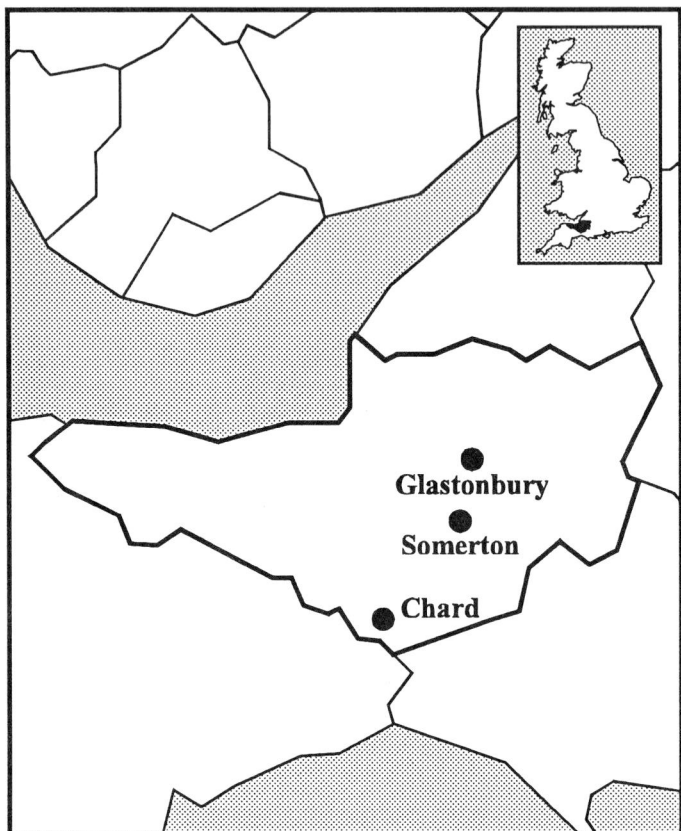

CHARD MUSEUM

GODWORTHY HOUSE
HIGH STREET
CHARD
SOMERSET

TELEPHONE: 0460-65091
OPEN: MONDAY - SATURDAY .... 10.30 - 4.30
                EARLY MAY TO MID OCTOBER
                PLUS SUNDAYS IN JULY & AUGUST
ADMISSION: CHARGE
SHOP. TOILETS.

   ♿   DISABLED ACCESS TO GROUND FLOOR.

The town of Chard was founded by Jocelyn, Bishop of Bath in 1235 and, after early success as a good market town, it changed its exports from wool to the finished broad cloth and in the 19th century was a mill town for plain net (lace). In the last 100 years engineering became the main industry, and more recently, food processing. These activities together with agricultural implements, a blacksmith's forge, carpenter's and wheelright's shops, and a 1940's garage are well displayed in this active local museum.

Two local celebrities also have a place in the museum. John Stringfellow, the pioneer of powered flight with his tools and models of his planes, and James Gillingham, pioneer of artificial limbs.

In 1863 Will Singleton, gamekeeper, had his arm shattered by the ramrod when firing a cannon in celebration of the Prince of Wales's marriage. It was amputated at the shoulder socket. A later conversation with James Gillingham, the local shoemaker, resulted in Gillingham making and fitting an artificial arm that was so good that Singleton could "lift a hundredweight or more, load and wheel a barrow.". The success was noted by the local doctor, Dr. Spicer, who induced Gillingham to show his skills in London. He became so popular that he gave up shoemaking and "threw his whole energy into this new sphere of usefulness." By 1903 he claimed to have treated over 7,000 patients; Sidney his son and later his grandson Geoffrey maintained the family connection until 1950 when the business passed to other hands and was closed in the 1960's. On display are some of the exquisitely made wooden articulated hands, boots, metal alloy limbs, legs with articulated feet, photographs and the tools and lathes used by James Gillingham.

SOMERSET RURAL LIFE MUSEUM

ABBEY FARM
CHILKWELL STREET
GLASTONBURY
SOMERSET

TELEPHONE: 0458-32903
OPEN: MONDAY - FRIDAY ....10.00 - 5.00
              SATURDAY & SUNDAY ....2.00 - 6.00
              1ST APRIL - 31ST OCTOBER
              MONDAY - FRIDAY ....10.00 - 5.00
              SATURDAY...1.00 - 4.00
              1ST NOVEMBER - 31ST MARCH
ADMISSION: CHARGE
SHOP. REFRESHMENTS (APRIL - SEPTEMBER).
TOILETS. SPECIAL ACTIVITIES.

DISABLED ACCESS TO GROUND FLOOR AND OUT
BUILDINGS.

PARTY BOOKINGS BY APPOINTMENT.

Opening to the public in 1976 at the Abbey Farm the following five years saw the repair of the farmhouse, buildings and magnificent Abbey Barn as a suitable place to display the collections illustrating the way of life of the rural community of Somerset. In the farmhouse the kitchen recaptures the atmosphere of the 1890's, while upstairs the life of one farm worker, John Hodges (1828-91), is told from the cradle to the grave with documents from the parish records, objects and photographs. Some of the items on display include a china slipper bedpan, Nelson's inhaler, china medicine cup and the 'hernia tree'. This is the trunk of an ash tree widened with wedges to a certain length to create a fissure. At dawn a suffering child was passed, feet first, through the fissure from East to West. A girl passed the child to a boy 3 times, the wedges were removed and the fissure plastered with clay. If the tree recovered and flourished a cure would be expected. A newspaper cutting of 1899 shows this cure was still in use then.

The farm buildings show local industries such as willow basket making, peat digging, cider making, marketing and a collection of agricultural implements and wagons. Outside are hens, sheep and geese and also a display of veterinary instruments.

Nearby is the Chalice Well, a place of legend, symbolism and atmosphere, whose chalybeate water is still used by many as a cure for asthma and arthritis. In 1751 even the King's Evil, blindness, ulcers and deafness were claimed to have been cured.

LYTES CARY MANOR

CHARLTON MACKRELL
SOMERTON
SOMERSET TA11 7HU

(␨) TELEPHONE: 0985-847 777 (GENERAL ENQUIRIES)
OPEN: MONDAY, WEDNESDAY & SATURDAY........2.00 - 6.00
.... OR DUSK IF EARLIER
1ST APRIL - 31 OCTOBER
ADMISSION: CHARGE. NATIONAL TRUST.
PLANTS FOR SALE.

& DISABLED ACCESS TO GARDEN ONLY.

The ancient manor of Lytes Carey was the home of the Lyte family from the 13th to the 18th centuries. It was Henry Lyte who published the Niewe Herball in 1578, a translation from the Flemish of Dodens, and dedicated to Queen Elisabeth "from my poore house at Lytescarie". A copy of the herbal is on display in the Great Hall with the pages turned regularly to show a different botanical drawing.

The garden has long paved walks, an orchard, a yew hedged alley leading to a formal pool and a border along the South Front, stocked with species of plants which were cultivated when Henry Lyte published his Niewe Herball.

Staffordshire

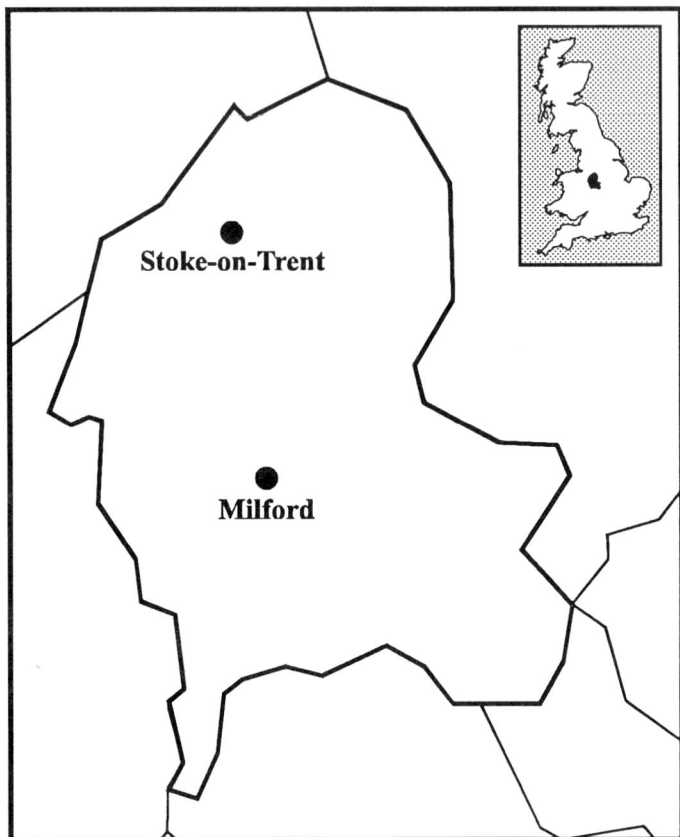

SHUGBOROUGH

MILFORD
NEAR STAFFORD
STAFFORDSHIRE ST17 0XB

TELEPHONE: 0889-881 388
OPEN: MONDAY - SUNDAY .... 11.00 - 5.00
             END MARCH - 30 OCTOBER
ADMISSION: CHARGE
N.T. MEMBERS FREE ENTRY TO MANSION HOUSE ONLY.
SHOP. REFRESHMENTS. TOILETS.

   ♿   DISABLED ACCESS TO MUSEUM AND FARM - APPOINTMENT
       FOR ACCESS TO GROUND FLOOR OF HOUSE.

   👫   HOUSE, MUSEUM, FARM & GARDENS OPEN 10.30 ALL YEAR
       TO BOOKED PARTIES.
       GUIDED TOURS FOR SCHOOL PARTIES. PICNIC AREA.

The Shugborough Estate is being restored as a 19th century working estate. The Hall is the 18th century home of the Earls of Lichfield and has a fine collection of French and English china, silver, paintings and furniture. In the stable block is the Staffordshire County's Museum with re-creations of 19th century servant life - a laundry, kitchens, working brew-house and medical gallery. Here a working display illustrates some of the techniques used by the traditional pharmacist with fittings from a nearby shop. There is also much information on the wall boards about Herbalism, the development of Pharmacy, Homeopathy, Astrology and Phlebotomy. The Victorian surgery has an operating table, similar to an ordinary scrubbed pine kitchen table but with the addition of some leather straps to hold the patient down. Surgical instruments include those associated with the head, amputations and the ear, nose and throat. General nursing techniques, midwifery and urine testing are also shown.

STAFFORD CITY MUSEUM & ART GALLERY

       BETHESDA STREET
       HANLEY
       STOKE-ON-TRENT
       STAFFORDSHIRE ST1 3DE

   ☎   TELEPHONE: 0782-202 173
       OPEN: MONDAY - SATURDAY.................................10.00 - 5.00
                      SUNDAY...2.00 - 5.00
       ADMISSION: FREE
       SHOP. REFRESHMENTS. TOILETS.

   ♿   DISABLED ACCESS TO WHOLE MUSEUM.

A purpose built museum housing not only one of the most important collections of English pottery and porcelain, especially Staffordshire, but displays ranging from archaeology and natural history to a Spitfire (the designer lived locally). Sant's Chemist Shop formerly sited on Market Street, Longton, features original mahogany and mirror-finish fittings taken from the shop in the early 1970's. These are fitted out with a variety of bottles, scales, measures, mortars and pestles, a weighing machine and equipment and materials associated with a dispensing chemist.

In addition to the material in the gallery, there is a substantial amount held in storage which is available for study by visitors, by appointment.

Suffolk

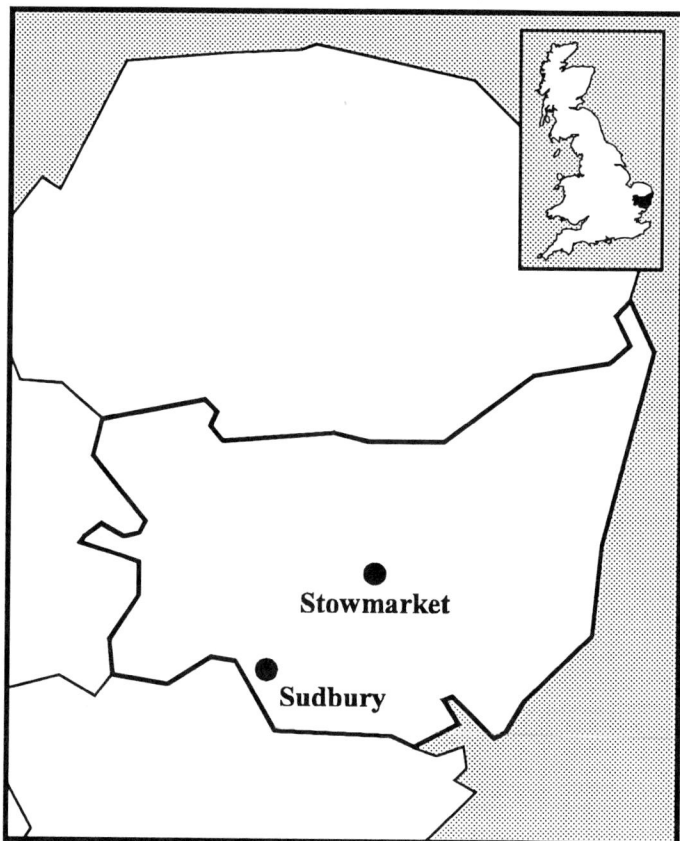

MUSEUM OF EAST ANGLIAN LIFE

STOWMARKET
SUFFOLK IP14 1DL

TELEPHONE: 0449-612 229
OPEN: MONDAY - SUNDAY ....10.00 - 5.00
1ST APRIL - 31ST OCTOBER
ADMISSION: CHARGE
SHOP. REFRESHMENTS. TOILETS.

DISABLED ACCESS TO ALL SITE.

GROUPS BY APPOINTMENT.

This attractively situated open air museum has re-constructed buildings which include a watermill, smithy and wind pump; craft workshops, industrial, domestic and agricultural displays and a working Suffolk Punch horse. The museum recently accepted part of the collection from the now closed St. Audry's Hospital, Melton, a large psychiatric institution and former County Asylum and Workhouse. The collection is mainly to do with the nursing of patients and the farm worked by the patients in the 19th century and early 20th century. It includes patients' and nurses' uniforms, a bed, crockery and cutlery and some farming equipment, but is not yet on display so please ring to make and appointment.

THE SUE RYDER MUSEUM

CAVENDISH
SUDBURY
SUFFOLK CO10 8AY

🕿 TELEPHONE: 0787-280 252
    OPEN: MONDAY - SATURDAY .... 10.00 - 5.30
                SUNDAY .... 10.00 - 11.00 & 12.30 - 5.30
    ADMISSION: CHARGE
    SHOP. REFRESHMENTS. TOILETS.
♿ DISABLED ACCESS.
🚶 GROUPS BY APPOINTMENT.

The Sue Ryder Foundation was formed in 1953 as a Living Memorial to those millions who died in two world wars, and to those who today are suffering and dying as a result of persecution. It is an international charity and seeks to fulfil its purpose regardless of race, religion or age. There are just over 80 homes in 14 countries, 24 of them in the United Kingdom.

This delightful museum depicts the work, background and history of the Foundation.

Surrey

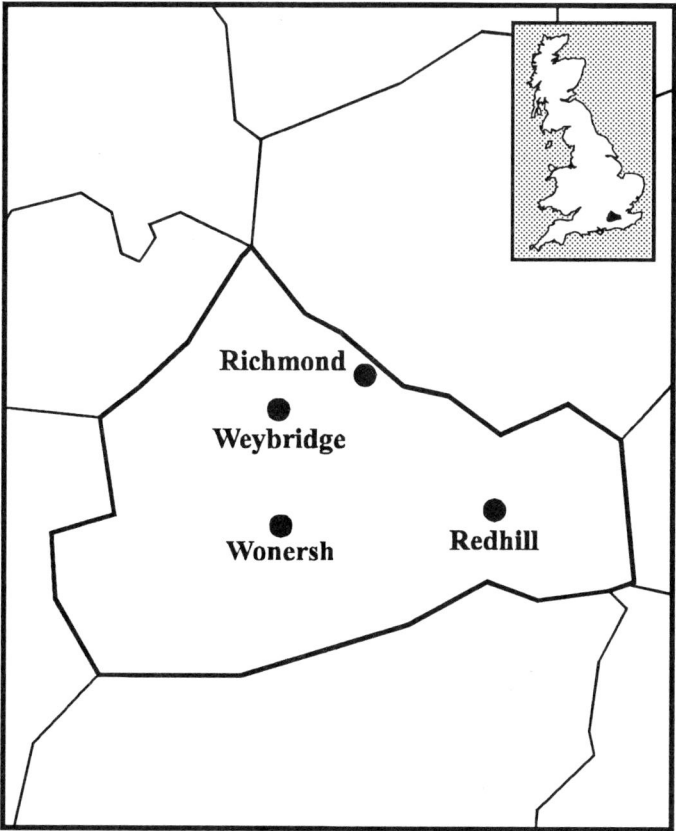

ROYAL EARLSWOOD HOSPITAL

BRIGHTON ROAD
REDHILL
SURREY RH1 6JL

☎ TELEPHONE: 0737-768 511 EXT. 8206
OPEN: BY APPOINTMENT

The hospital itself is due to close soon and the future of the museum is far from certain. It is hoped that it will be kept intact and not dispersed as it provides a unique record of the history of the hospital from its founding in 1847 to the present day. There are on display the Royal Charter, photographs, artefacts from the hospital including a crested washing bowl and soap dish, top hat, wooden leg and locks and lamps. Also scopes, sounds, orthopaedic instruments, syringes, a child's carriage, a book of cuttings from 1874 and assorted leaflets, musical instruments from 1910 and implements from the hospital farm. One of the most famous inmates was James Henry Pullen, a deaf idiot (possibly autistic savant), who made the most intricate large model ships. The Alexandra was a 40 gun man o' war and the ivory tusks used were donated by King Edward VII.

ROYAL BOTANIC GARDENS

KEW
RICHMOND
SURREY TW9 3AB

☎ TELEPHONE: 081-940 1171
OPEN: MONDAY - SUNDAY ....9.30 - 5.00
            LAST ADMISSION..4.30
GLASS HOUSES & GALLERIES....................................9.30 - 4.30
ADMISSION: CHARGE
SHOP. TOILETS. REFRESHMENTS.

&. DISABLED ACCESS.

👫 GUIDED TOURS FOR GROUPS BY ARRANGEMENT.

Princess Augusta, an enthusiastic gardener and mother of George III, first developed Kew as a botanic garden in 1759, with 9 acres laid out with walls, trees and herbaceous plants. Sir William Chambers designed many of the garden's 24 splendid buildings of which only the Pagoda and Orangery remain. George III joined the two former Royal estates of Richmond and Kew and with extra acquisitions the gardens now extend to 300 acres. The Palm House (designed by Decimus Burton and Richard Turner an ironmaster) was built to house the many exotic plants collected from China, Australia and Brazil.

To-day Kew is concerned with the conservation of all plants and has a continuing programme of research for crops economically and environmentally suitable for third world countries; research in developing new insecticides and medicines; their World Seed Bank, Library, Herbarium and Archive's constitute the world's finest botanical resource.

Kew Palace, originally built for a 17th century Dutch merchant, has a garden laid out in design and planting of that period. In the sunken herb and nosegay garden are many well labelled medicinal plants. The 'uses' are taken from Gerard's Herbal, 1597; Parkinson's Theatrum Botanicum, 1640; and Turner's New Herbal, 1551. These include comfrey for a pain in the back; yellow asphodel for coughs; salvia for the eyes; artemesia for pimples; red germane for inward bleeding; marsh mallow for stones and gravel and acanthus for gout, burns and scalds.

DE TREY, DENTSPLY

HAMM MOOR LANE
ADDLESTONE
WEYBRIDGE
SURREY KT15 2SE

☎ TELEPHONE: 0932-853 422
OPEN: BY APPOINTMENT ONLY FOR SERIOUS
         RESEARCHERS.

The company supplies dental equipment to the trade but does have a collection of dental instruments, mostly hand instruments with some laboratory items dating from the late 18th century. Not normally available to members of the public but in special cases it would be opened to serious researchers.

THE BRITISH RED CROSS SOCIETY

ARCHIVES SECTION
BARNETT HILL
WONERSH
GUILDFORD
SURREY GU5 0RF

☎ TELEPHONE: 0483-898 595
OPEN: BY APPOINTMENT ONLY

The Red Cross movement was founded in 1863 at a meeting in Geneva which, in the following year, was formalised by the signing of the First Geneva Convention. The meeting had been held following the publication in 1862 of Henry Dunant's book which recorded his experiences, as a civilian, at the Battle of Solferino in 1859 when there were 40,000 casualties in only 16 hours. He urged governments to help the sick and wounded in war of both sides in addition to the military medical attention they might receive. Individual countries were encouraged to set up their own national Red Cross societies, the British being founded in 1870 known as the British National Society for Aid to the Sick and Wounded in War. In 1905 it became the British Red Cross Society.

The museum provides a comprehensive look at Red Cross activities from 1859 to the present day. The display consists principally of photographs, uniforms, medals, postcards, medical and nursing equipment and embroideries, including the Changi quilt worked by the women internees of Changi Gaol, Singapore early in 1942.

The Society's records date from 1870 with official reports on its activities in the Franco-Prussian War of 1870/71. Record cards are held for WW1 and WW2 VAD's and these include such famous names as Vera Brittain, John Masefield, Freya Stark and Agatha Christie. In addition there is a reference library and extensive photographic collection.

The Archive Section is at the top of the former home of the Thomas Cook family which, having been used as a hospital during the war, was handed over to the Red Cross in 1944. The large house and beautiful grounds are now used as a training centre for Red Cross trainers and as a residential conference centre available to any business organisation.

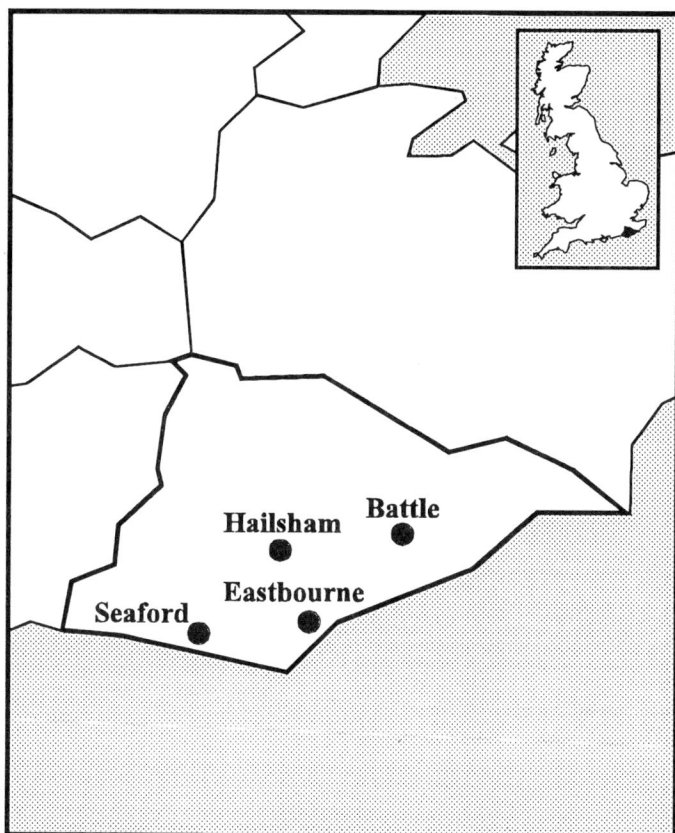

BUCKLEYS MUSEUM OF SHOPS

90 HIGH STREET
BATTLE
NR. HASTINGS
EAST SUSSEX TN33 0AQ

TELEPHONE: 04246-4269
OPEN: MONDAY - SUNDAY ....10.00 - 5.30
           EXTENDED OPENING IN JUNE, JULY & AUGUST
           JANUARY - MARCH SUBJECT TO CHANGE
ADMISSION: CHARGE
SHOP. REFRESHMENTS. TOILETS.

 & DISABLED ACCESS.

Started as a hobby by Mrs. Annette Buckley in 1972 this family concern now housed in the old Wealden Hall, evokes a 100 years of nostalgia with exhibits from 1850-1950. A pre-war grocer's shop, village post-office, pub, boot repairer, draper and outfitters, lace maker, pawnbroker, toy shop and ironmonger together with the chemist are crammed with fascinating stock. The chemist, K.H. Emeleus, is named after a local chemist, established in Battle over 200 years ago and displays a fascinating collection of remedies and patent medicines.

MUSEUM OF SHOPS & SOCIAL HISTORY

> 20 CORNFIELD TERRACE
> EASTBOURNE
> EAST SUSSEX BN21 4NS

 Ⓢ TELEPHONE: 0323-37143
OPEN: MONDAY - SUNDAY .... 10.00 - 5.30
CLOSED: JANUARY & FIRST WEEK FEBRUARY
            & WINTER MONTHS 5.00
ADMISSION: CHARGE
TOILETS. SHOP. TEA SHOP NEARBY.

 & DISABLED ACCESS GROUND FLOOR ONLY.

A husband and wife team have spent 30 years collecting over 35,000 exhibits which have been laid out on three floors of authentic old shops and displays to capture uniquely the atmosphere of 100 years of social history (1850-1950). The grocer sells biscuits from glass-topped jars, the draper displays lace, clothes and hats and the toy shop trains, soldiers and puzzles. The chemist, Mr. Cure-All, dispenses his medicines from a vast array of pills and potions which line the shelves in glass jars and cardboard boxes.

MICHELHAM PRIORY

UPPER DICKER
NR. HAILSHAM
EAST SUSSEX BN27 3QS

☎ TELEPHONE: 0323-844 224
    OPEN: MONDAY - SUNDAY ....11.00 - 5.30
              MID MARCH - END OCTOBER
              SUNDAY ONLY..11.00 - 4.00
              FEBRUARY, MARCH & NOVEMBER
    ADMISSION: CHARGE
    SHOP. REFRESHMENTS. TOILETS.
  ♿ DISABLED ACCESS TO GROUND FLOOR & GARDEN.

Situated at the head of the Cuckmere valley the site was chosen for an Augustinian priory in the 13th century and became part of the religious life of the time. After the dissolution of the monasteries it was used as a farmhouse. Today the monastic rooms and Tudor room can be visited together with two exhibition rooms. Outside the buildings include a forge and wheelwright's museum and rope museum and watermill. On the south lawn is a monastic-style physic garden established in 1981, containing nearly 100 plants used in medieval times for medicinal and culinary purposes. The different herbs are planted in groups for treating the same disorder; stomach and liver; head, hair and skin; bites, stings, burns and poisons; wounds; depression, insomnia and nightmares; and childbirth and children's diseases.

SEAFORD MUSEUM OF LOCAL HISTORY

MARTELLO TOWER
NO 74 ESPLANADE
SEAFORD
EAST SUSSEX BN25 1TU

☎ TELEPHONE: 0323-899 007
    OPEN: WEDNESDAY & SATURDAY...........................2.30 - 4.30
              SUNDAY....................................11.00 - 1.00 & 2.30 - 4.30
              GOOD FRIDAY - MID OCTOBER
              SUNDAY ONLY.........................11.00 - 1.00 & 2.30 - 4.30
              WINTER.
              B.H. AS SUNDAY.

ADMISSION: CHARGE. SPECIAL RATES FOR PARTIES BY
ARRANGEMENT.
SHOP. ADJACENT TOILETS ON PROMENADE.

Martello Tower No.74 is the most westerly of a chain of
103 similar fortifications running from Aldeburgh on the east
coast to Seaford on the south. Built in 1806 against a
threatened Napoleonic invasion, it has an original cannon on
its roof, and affords magnificent views over Seaford town
and bay.

The museum moved here in 1979 and is run entirely by
enthusiastic volunteers. Displays include shops, tableaux and
fascinating collections of material from prehistoric times to
the present day. The shops include a general store,
dressmaker's parlour, photographer, ironmonger, toy shop
and chemist. Also Victorian and wartime kitchens, Church
Street school, an agricultural scene and a model of the
railway station in 1922. There is an extensive library of
photographs, press cuttings and pictures. The chemist's shop
has a collection of bottles, jars and tins, inhalers, babies
bottles, instruments and enamel bowls from the 19th and 20th
centuries.

West Sussex

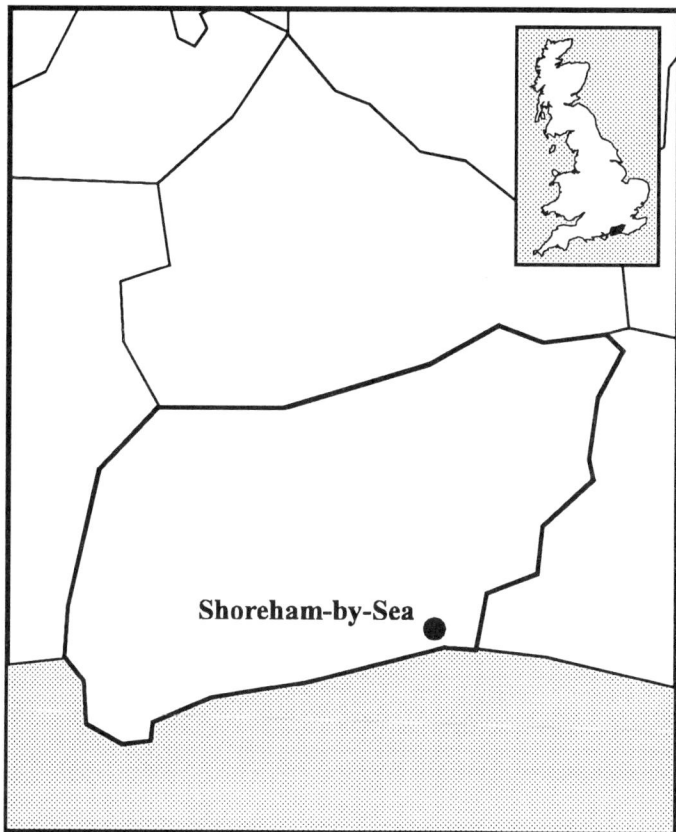

Shoreham-by-Sea

MARLIPINS MUSEUM

HIGH STREET
SHOREHAM-BY-SEA
WEST SUSSEX BN4 5NN

☎ TELEPHONE: 0273-462 994
OPEN: TUESDAY - SATURDAY .... 10.00 - 1.00 & 2.00 - 4.30
            MAY - SEPTEMBER
            SUNDAY...2.00 - 4.30
ADMISSION: FREE, DONATIONS APPRECIATED
SHOP.

 ♿   DISABLED ACCESS VERY DIFFICULT OWING TO NATURE OF BUILDING.

The building was constructed in Norman times and later, and was possibly built as a customs house. It has an interesting chequer-work facade of knapped flint and Caen stone. It now contains a museum of Shoreham's local, industrial and maritime history, including a gallery housing an attractive collection of pictures, photographs and postcards of local interest. Amongst the maritime items is a ship surgeon's set of instruments. Lined with blue velvet it contains 4 curved steel stitching needles, steel bladed double toothed saw with ebony handle, 7 ebony handled instruments including scalpels and a curved blunted probe with needle eye in the end of the blade. Also double ended tweezers, brass screw tourniquet and several long gut rods.

Tyne & Wear

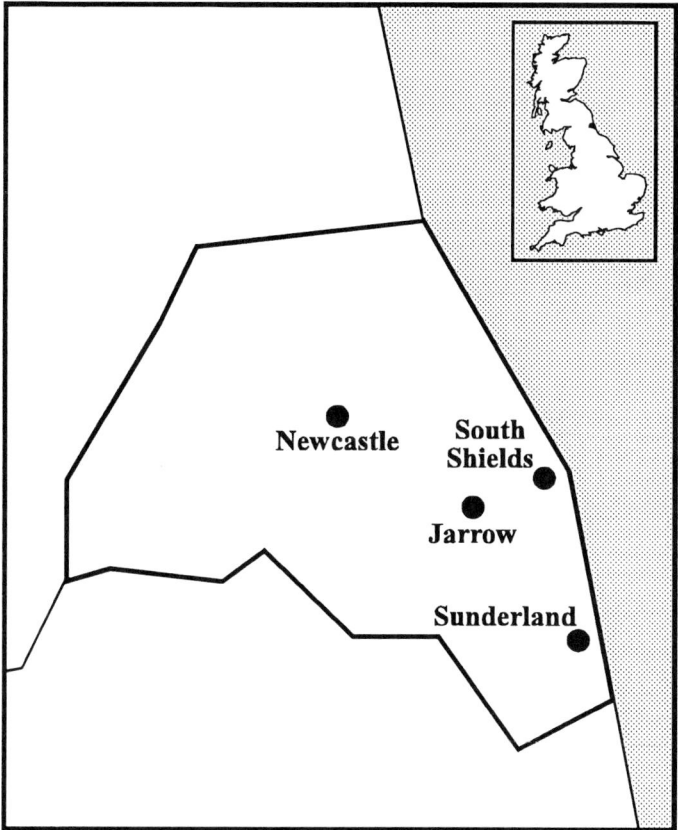

THE BEDE MONASTERY MUSEUM

JARROW HALL
CHURCH BANK
JARROW
TYNE & WEAR NE32 3DY

☎ TELEPHONE: 091-489 2106
OPEN: TUESDAY - SATURDAY ....10.00 - 5.30
SUNDAY...2.30 - 5.30
1ST APRIL - 31ST OCTOBER
TUESDAY - SATURDAY ....11.00 - 4.30
SUNDAY...2.30 - 5.30
1ST NOVEMBER - 31ST MARCH

OPEN BANK HOLIDAY MONDAYS
ADMISSION: CHARGE
CRAFT SHOP. REFRESHMENTS. TOILETS.

  ♿   DISABLED ACCESS TO GROUND FLOOR & GARDEN.

  🚶   GROUPS TO PRE-BOOK.

The museum tells the story of the monastery of St. Paul, Jarrow, home of the Venerable Bede (A.D. 673-735), the foremost scholar of his age and the author of many books, most notably 'The Ecclesiastical History of the English People'. The monastery has been excavated and many finds - the earliest coloured window glass in the country, sculpture, building materials, metalwork and pottery - are displayed alongside a model of the 8th century monastery. In 1982 a herb garden was established, one part based on the raised beds of the 16th and 17th centuries and the second on the long narrow beds as recommended in the St. Gall monastic ideal plan (c. A.D. 816). The medicinal plants include hyssop, valerian, periwinkle, skirret, bistort, toadflax, lungwort, buglos, comfrey and Roman wormwood. The next project is the reconstruction of an Anglo-Saxon farm.

MUSEUM OF SCIENCE & ENGINEERING

BLANDFORD HOUSE
BLANDFORD SQUARE
NEWCASTLE
TYNE AND WEAR NE1 4JA

  ☉   TELEPHONE: 091-232 6789
        OPEN: TUESDAY - FRIDAY......................................10.00 - 5.30
                  SATURDAY...10.00 - 4.30
        ADMISSION: FREE
        SHOP. REFRESHMENTS. TOILETS.

  ♿   DISABLED ACCESS TO WHOLE MUSEUM.

The early 19th century building was once the headquarters of the Co-operative Wholesale Society but is now dedicated to the engineering, mining, shipbuilding and science of Newcastle. There are galleries on motor power from steam to petrol, maritime achievements, pioneers of industry including Swan, Stevenson and Armstrong; the

Tyne tunnel showing the history of Newcastle from the Romans to the 1960's and a 'Science Factory' for children.

Surgical and dental instruments belonging to the Newcastle Company of Barber-Surgeons, a 19th century operating table and treatment chair, 1930's dental instruments, miscellaneous instruments from a local general practitioner (1930-1960) and a 1950 iron-lung machine, make an interesting medical collection. The social history gallery has a display on the advent of the NHS and the department of child health. The exhibition area has changing displays which often include medical items. A small amount of related material is in the reserve collection, available by appointment.

ARBEIA ROMAN FORT & MUSEUM

BARING STREET
SOUTH SHIELDS
TYNE AND WEAR NE33 2BB

○ TELEPHONE: 091-454 4093
OPEN: GROUNDS & GARDEN
               MONDAY - FRIDAY ....10.00 - 5.30
               MUSEUM
               TUESDAY - FRIDAY ....10.00 - 5.30
               BOTH
               SATURDAY ....10.00 - 4.30
               SUNDAY...2.00 - 5.00
CLOSED: SUNDAY
               OCTOBER - EASTER
ADMISSION: FREE
SHOP.

& DISABLED ACCESS.

Built in the 1st and 2nd centuries A.D. the fort guarded the entrance to the river Tyne. In A.D. 208 it was converted into a supply base serving the large garrison of Hadrian's Wall and its vicinity. Later extensive rebuilding saw a large courtyard residence for a senior official and it is probable that the Roman occupation continued until the 5th century. The West gate has been reconstructed and a museum houses the many finds including some tombstones, a dedication slab marking the introduction of the water supply in A.D. 222, some cremations and skulls from the cemetery, and items illustrating the day to day life of the soldiers in the garrison. A Roman Garden has recently been planted, although no such garden existed at South Shields, to display the plants used in the kitchens; such as herbs, fruit and vegetables and staple cereals, those used for rituals, festivals, and garlands, and medicinal plants. The latter includes soapwort, squill, tansy, rosa gallica, Spanish broom, marigold, rue and camomile for use as either a stimulant, laxative, painkiller, treatment or cure.

GRINDON MUSEUM

GRINDON LANE
SUNDERLAND
TYNE & WEAR

☎ TELEPHONE: 091-514 1235
OPEN: MONDAY & FRIDAY .... 9.30 - 12.30 & 1.30 - 6.00
TUESDAY & WEDNESDAY .... 9.30 - 12.30 & 1.30 - 5.00
SATURDAY .... 9.30 - 12.15 & 1.15 - 4.00
SUNDAY .... 2.00 - 5.00
JUNE - SEPTEMBER
ADMISSION: FREE
SHOP. TOILETS. REFRESHMENTS.

Edwardian Sunderland is brought to life in what was once a ship-builder's house. There are lavish period room displays of a kitchen, nursery, sitting room, chemist's shop and dentist's surgery. The chemist has a drug run, bottles, jars and boxes of patent medicines, a pestle and mortar and a water filter amongst other pill making equipment. The dentist uses a foot-operated drill and has a wide range of teeth extracting forceps.

SUNDERLAND MUSEUM & ART GALLERY

BOROUGH ROAD
SUNDERLAND
TYNE & WEAR SR1 1PP

☎ TELEPHONE: 091-514 1235
OPEN: TUESDAY - FRIDAY .... 10.00 - 5.30

SATURDAY ....10.00 - 4.00
SUNDAY...2.00 - 5.00
ADMISSION: FREE
SHOP. REFRESHMENTS. TOILETS.
 ♿ DISABLED ACCESS.

Sharing the same building as the Central Library in the town centre the museum graphically displays the history of Wearside from pre-history to to-day. Local lustreware pottery and the revolutionary 'Pyrex', shipbuilding, live exhibits in the wildlife gallery, the paintings of L.S. Lowry and Edward Burra and others make this an exciting and diverse museum. A display on the 1831 cholera epidemic in Sunderland includes a couple of rare prints as well as a portrait of Dr. Clanny, one of the pioneering doctors involved in treating the disease. He was also involved in the development of the miners safety lamp, which was to become so important in this coal mining region.

Warwickshire

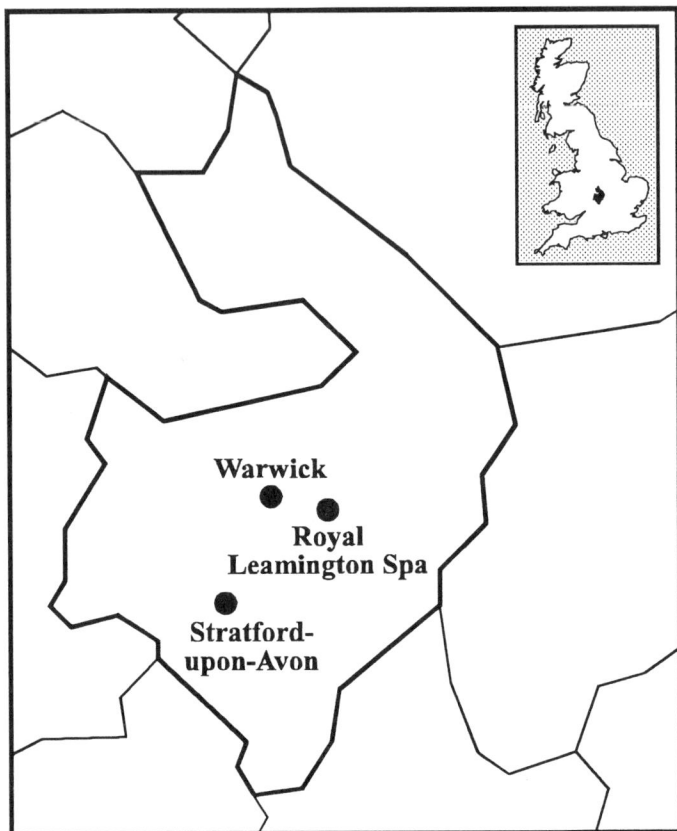

ART GALLERY & MUSEUM

AVENUE ROAD
ROYAL LEAMINGTON SPA
WARWICKSHIRE

☎ TELEPHONE 0926-426 559
OPEN: MONDAY - SATURDAY .... 10.00 - 1.00 & 2.00 - 5.00
              THURSDAY EVENING.................................... 6.00 - 8.00
CLOSED: WEDNESDAY
ADMISSION: FREE
SHOP.

♿ DISABLED ACCESS TO ALL MUSEUM.

Queen Victoria gave the resort its Royal title when she claimed it was her 'favourite town' for drinking the waters. It was in 1586 that a salty underground spring was first discovered and another 200 years before it developed into a fashionable spa town. By the middle of the 19th century Dr. Jephson achieved fame and fortune with his medical treatments.

The museum has a social history room showing the rise of the town's popularity as a spa. The art gallery has a collection of 17th and 18th century Dutch paintings, works by local artists and galleries for temporary exhibitions. The mineral rich waters are available from a public tap set on the bridge near the Pump Rooms - bring your own bottle!

HALL'S CROFT

> OLD TOWN
> STRATFORD-UPON-AVON
> WARWICKSHIRE CV37 6QW

☎ TELEPHONE: 0789-204 016 (BIRTHPLACE TRUST)
    OPEN: MONDAY - SATURDAY...................................9.30 - 5.30
                SUNDAY...10.30 - 5.00
                1ST MARCH - 30TH OCTOBER
                MONDAY - SATURDAY................................10.00 - 4.00
                SUNDAY...1.30 - 4.00
                1ST NOVEMBER - 28TH FEBRUARY
    ADMISSION: CHARGE, (& COMBINED TICKET FOR ALL
    5 SHAKESPEARE PLACES)
    SHOP. REFRESHMENTS. TOILETS.

 ♿ DISABLED ACCESS TO GROUND FLOOR AND GARDENS.

Hall's Croft is the outstanding half-timbered home of Shakespeare's daughter, Susanna, and her husband Dr. John Hall from 1607 - 1616. Dr. Hall built up a large and fashionable medical practice not only in the town but in the neighbouring counties, where he attended many noble families. A selection from his case-books, which was published in 1657, throws some interesting sidelights on the doctor and his patients and is on display in the house, together with a letter from an aggrieved patient upbraiding the Doctor for not hastening immediately to his bedside when summoned! The Dispensary is furnished in the style of a contemporary consulting-room, complete with apothecaries' jars for medicines, herbs and pills, herbals and pestles and mortars. Upstairs the long Upper Hall has a display of 19th century medical equipment, references to medicine in Shakespeare's works, and a display of disease and plague and the influence of Van Leeuwenhoek and his invention of the microscope. The charming walled garden is planted with roses, herbaceous flowers and herbs which may have been used by Dr. Hall in his medicines.

WARWICKSHIRE MUSEUM

MARKET SQUARE
WARWICK
WARWICKSHIRE CV34 4SA

ⓓ TELEPHONE: 0926-410 410 EXT. 2500
OPEN: MONDAY - SATURDAY .... 10.00 - 5.30
              SUNDAY .... 2.30 - 5.00
          MAY - SEPTEMBER ONLY
ADMISSION: FREE
SHOP.

In the centre of the town in the old Market Hall the museum displays the history of Warwickshire with a strong emphasis on archaeology, geology and wild life including the giant fossil plesiosaur and the Sheldon tapestry map. Held in the reserve collection and available by appointment with the curator of Social History are some boxes of medical instruments, pill-rolling equipment, cupping sets and amputation sets.

West Midlands

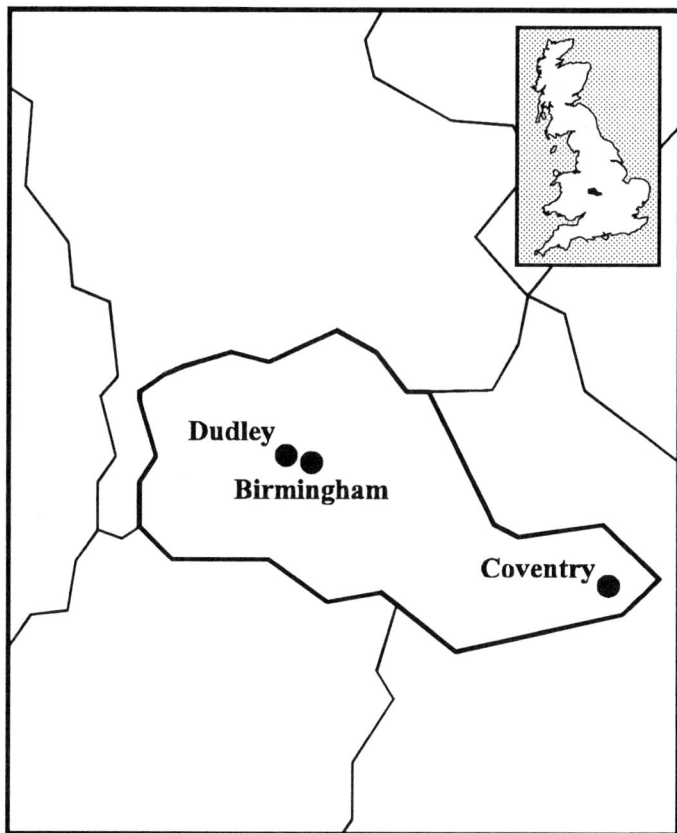

BIRMINGHAM MUSEUM OF SCIENCE & INDUSTRY

NEWHALL STREET
BIRMINGHAM
WEST MIDLANDS B3 1RZ

☎ TELEPHONE: 021-235 1661
   OPEN: MONDAY - SATURDAY..................................9.30 - 5.00
                SUNDAY...2.00 - 5.00
   ADMISSION: FREE
   SHOP. TOILETS.

♿ DISABLED ACCESS TO ALL FLOORS.

The museum has a wide range of industrial items including steam engines, machine tools, small arms, different forms of transport and scientific instruments. Amongst these is a Danatome Tomography Unit. This was manufactured by Philips Electrical Company in 1954 and was developed from a prototype built around 1946 to increase the diagnostic value of x-rays. This equipment gave close control over the penetrating depth of rays enabling photographs to be taken at various layers through the body to help locate affected areas. This machine was in use at East Birmingham Hospital until 1985 when it was replaced by a more modern 'Scanner'.

Other displays include the music room, pen collection, domestic and communications equipment, arms and cycles and a series of replica workshops. The new Light on Science exhibition is a 'hands on' exploration of light, sound, bridges, gyroscopes and pendulums.

MUSEUM OF BRITISH ROAD TRANSPORT

ST. AGNES LANE
HALES STREET
COVENTRY
WEST MIDLANDS CV1 1PN

℡ TELEPHONE: 0203-832 425
OPEN: MONDAY - SUNDAY .... 10.00 - 5.00
           EXCEPT XMAS DAY & BOXING DAY
ADMISSION: CHARGE
TOILETS. SHOP.

&. DISABLED ACCESS AND TOILET.

The largest display of British made road transport under one roof includes Edwardian and vintage vehicles set in period streets and the development of the family car through the 1930's, 40's and 50's to the latest luxury Jaguar. Bicycles and motorcycles, buses and commercial vehicles are displayed with some late 1950's and early 60's ambulances together with a wide range of equipment and accessories.

THE BLACK COUNTRY MUSEUM

TIPTON ROAD
DUDLEY
WEST MIDLANDS DY1 4SQ

① TELEPHONE: 021-557 9643
OPEN: MONDAY - SUNDAY ....10.00 - 5.00
CLOSED: AT DUSK IN WINTER
ADMISSION: CHARGE
SHOP. REFRESHMENTS.

& DISABLED ACCESS TO GROUND FLOOR SITES, ARCHIVE
CENTRE AND LIBRARY.

🖈 BOOKED PARTIES FREE GUIDED TOUR.

Established in 1975 as a charitable company the Museum is concerned with the preservation and care of buildings and machinery that are fast becoming redundant in the Black Country. Set on a 26-acre site with as many working exhibits as possible, costumed demonstrators re-create the living and working conditions of the last century. A 1920 single-deck electric tramcar runs between the entrance and the village passing the replica Newcomen Engine of 1712 and the colliery of the 1850's, where an underground visit can be made 'Into the Thick'. Normally the Glass cutter, Chain maker, Brass founder or Boat builder are on hand, and the narrow boats will take visitors into the Dudley Tunnel to the spectacular Singing Cavern. In the Village the chemist's shop is housed in a replica building based on the premises of Mr. Harold Emile Doo of Netherton in 1882. The fittings and fixtures are original Victorian combined with a vast array of 1930's and 1940's stock. The 'shop assistants' will demonstrate pill rolling on a brass and mahogany pill-making machine and provide information on the shop.

Wiltshire

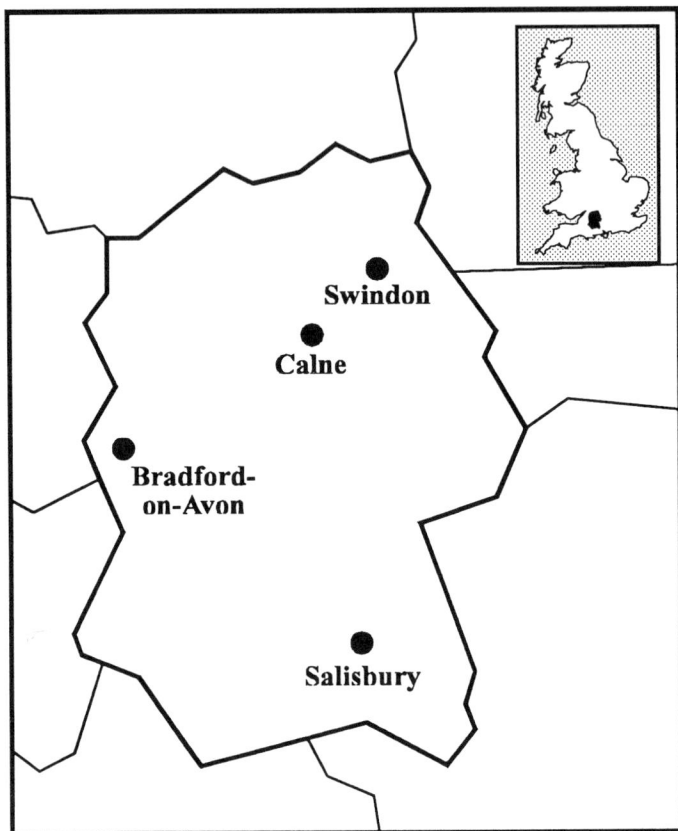

BRADFORD ON AVON MUSEUM

BRIDGE STREET
BRADFORD ON AVON
WILTSHIRE

TELEPHONE: 02216-3280
OPEN: WEDNESDAY - FRIDAY ....2.00 - 4.00
                SATURDAY..10.30 - 4.00
                SUNDAY ....2.00 - 4.00
ADMISSION: FREE

DISABLED ACCESS.

The museum is run by volunteers of the Bradford on Avon Museum Society, sited in the new library, and has amongst much fascinating material a pharmacy that has been in the town since 1863. The last owner, Richard Thorney Christopher, bought the shop in 1908, after travelling in Singapore and India. Having gained a taste for curries in the East he was soon selling his own powder mixes as well as a range of eastern inspired perfumes and beauty preparations. The shop has a mahogany counter, shelves, cabinets, dispensary and drug run which displays the glass bottles, some with their original contents, carboys and some laboratory glassware. Also a wide range of pharmacy equipment, stock items including old packages of medicines, cleaners, some surgical and veterinary equipment, photographic equipment, Christopher's travelling medicine case complete with contents which he acquired in India, and the complete run of prescription books from 1863 to 1986.

BOWOOD HOUSE & GARDENS

CALNE
WILTSHIRE

☎ TELEPHONE: 0249-812 102
OPEN: MONDAY - SUNDAY ....11.00 - 6.00 OR DUSK
         1ST APRIL - 1ST NOVEMBER
ADMISSION: CHARGE
SHOP. PLANT CENTRE. REFRESHMENTS. TOILETS.
ADVENTURE PLAYGROUND.

 ♿ DISABLED ACCESS TO GROUND FLOOR.

 ⅄ GROUPS BY ARRANGEMENT.

The 'Big House' of 1725 was constantly changed and re-modelled by Henry Keene and Robert Adam before being finally demolished in 1955. To-day the present Lord and Lady Shelburne live in the 'Little House', the Adam wing and courts, which enables them to keep the park, pleasure grounds and estate as a beautiful and rewarding heritage for the future.

The extensive and well cared for gardens provide a lovely setting for the house. Entering by the Orangery which has a collection of sculpture, at the end on the left is a small room called the laboratory. It was in this room that Dr. Joseph Priestley in August 1774 discovered oxygen. He was librarian and tutor to the first Lord Lansdowne's sons and worked at Bowood from 1773-1780. The room has letters from Priestley, a photograph and engraving of the apparatus and letters from Jeremy Bentham. The laboratory was also used by the scientist John Ingenhouse who discovered the process of photosynthesis and helped to pioneer an inoculation against smallpox.

The house has also a Robert Adam library, chapel, Georgian exhibition room with costumed figures, cases of heirlooms and jewel room.

SALISBURY & SOUTH WILTSHIRE MUSEUM

THE KING'S HOUSE
65 THE CLOSE
SALISBURY
WILTSHIRE SP1 2EN

☎ TELEPHONE: 0722-332 151
OPEN: MONDAY - SATURDAY .... 10.00 - 5.00
          SUNDAY .... 2.00 - 5.00
          JULY & AUGUST ONLY & TWO WEEKS OF
          SALISBURY FESTIVAL IN EARLY SEPTEMBER
ADMISSION: CHARGE
SHOP. REFRESHMENTS. TOILETS.
♿ DISABLED ACCESS TO GROUND FLOOR.

The King's House, a fine Grade 1 listed building, was originally the Salisbury residence of the abbots of Sherborne but, after the Reformation, the house was leased to secular tenants and visits by James I led to its being named the King's House. In 1978, after the closure of the Diocesan Training College (1851), the museum purchased the lease and moved in during 1981. Now it is one of the nation's most important archaeological museums drawing on its rich local historical sites. Local history, ceramics and glass, pictures, costumes, Salisbury's crafts and industries, and a 1930's doctor's surgery make a fascinating collection. The surgery is that of Dr. Philip Neighbour of Amesbury and illustrates well the 'sparse' conditions in which many doctors worked.

LYDIARD HOUSE & PARK

LYDIARD TREGOZE
SWINDON
WILTSHIRE SN5 9PA

☎ TELEPHONE: 0793-770 401
OPEN: MONDAY - SATURDAY........... 10.00 - 1.00 & 2.00 - 5.30
              SUNDAY...2.00 - 5.30
ADMISSION: FREE
SHOP. REFRESHMENTS & TOILETS IN VISITORS CENTRE IN THE PARK.

& DISABLED ACCESS TO GROUND FLOOR.

Lydiard was mentioned in the Doomsday Book and after a series of descents and marriages passed into the hands of the St. John family who were to hold it for 500 years until 1940. Henry St. John, well known Tory statesman and political philosopher, was created Viscount Bolingbroke for his services as Secretary of State to Queen Anne. The property was purchased by Swindon Corporation in 1943 and the house has been painstakingly restored to its former glory with some fine classical and rococo ceilings and a painted glass window. It houses a fine display of furniture and a notable collection of St. John family portraits.

The medical items, which can be seen by appointment, include 19th century glass medicine bottles and jars; a glass measuring jar and cylinder; wood and glass syringes; Dr. Ward's ointment introducer; pill boxes, tins and embrocation tins; a metal spatula, and a round ebony box with a label indicating pastilles, as recommended by Sarah Bernhardt, Ellen Terry and Sir Henry Irving.

THE GREAT WESTERN RAILWAY MUSEUM

FARRINGDON ROAD
SWINDON
WILTSHIRE SN1 5BJ

☎ TELEPHONE: 0793-493 189
    OPEN: MONDAY - SATURDAY .... 10.00 - 5.00
                SUNDAY .... 2.00 - 5.00
                LAST ADMISSION 4.30
    ADMISSION: CHARGE
    SHOP.

♧ DISABLED ACCESS TO GROUND FLOOR TO VIEW
    LOCOMOTIVES.

The G.W.R. Museum is set in the heart of Brunel's railway village, and the exhibits celebrate the glories of 'God's Wonderful Railway'. Housed in a building which was once a Wesleyan Chapel, 5 locomotives dominate the main hall, including the replica Broad Gauge engine 'North Star', and G.J. Churchward's 4-6-0 'Lode Star'. Next door, visitors can step back in time to visit a restored railwayman's cottage with many original fittings.

G.W.R. founded its own Medical Fund Society in 1847, when a rateable subscription was deducted each week from every man's wages. In 1869 it introduced revolutionary 'Washing, Turkish, Swimming and Shower Baths'. A hospital was opened in 1872, for accidents only, and was to be free for all members of the Society with other workers paying a small fee. In 1887 a dental clinic was opened and 5 years later new consulting rooms, waiting halls and a dispensary. By 1944 the hospital had an X-ray department, blood-donor service, an ophthalmic and physical medicine department, a minor operating theatre, chiropody department, and skin, psychological and paediatric clinics. Items from the medical fund on display include a mortar and pestle, two framed medical fund posters, combined scales and height measure, doctor's call box, commode, mirror, pharmacists' drug box, paperwork and medical fund chairman's chair. An artificial limb, of the type made in the trim shop, is also on display, for a worker unfortunate enough to lose one while in the company's service.

North Yorkshire

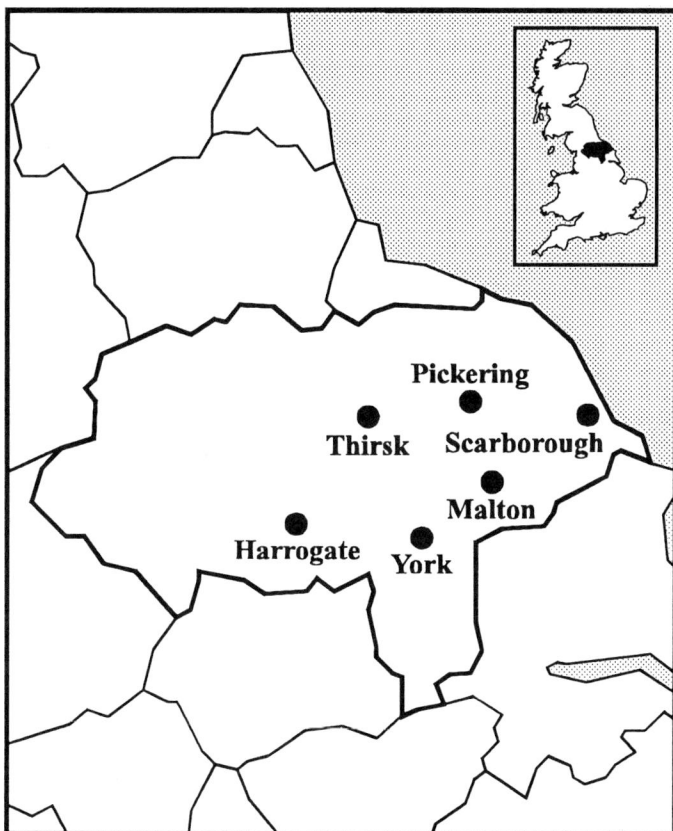

NIDDERDALE MUSEUM

THE COUNCIL OFFICES
PATELEY BRIDGE
HARROGATE
NORTH YORKSHIRE HG3 5AY

TELEPHONE: 0423-711 225
OPEN: MONDAY - SUNDAY ....2.00 - 5.00
         SUMMER ONLY
         SUNDAY...2.00 - 5.00
         OCTOBER - EASTER
ADMISSION: CHARGE
TOILETS. SHOP.

Founded in 1975 by a group of enthusiasts who realised that much of the life of the dale was quickly disappearing, the museum of nine rooms is in the old union workhouse. The rooms are devoted to leisure and religion, a collection of cameras, household crockery and equipment, transport, costumes, crafts and agriculture and a wide range of reconstructed shops. Amongst them is the chemist's shop with pill-making equipment, scales, measures, weights, patent medicines and an excellent range of drug and perfume bottles. Also a collection of dental instruments and some medical items donated by a local G.P. A brass enema and catheter set, each in its own travelling case, a monaural stethoscope and a fine bleeding set with an accompanying note 'Reputed to have belonged to Colonel Lane-Fox, physician to Charles II'.

ROYAL PUMP ROOM MUSEUM

CROWN PLACE
HARROGATE
NORTH YORKSHIRE HG1 2RY

☎ TELEPHONE: 0423-503 340
OPEN: TUESDAY - SATURDAY ....10.30 - 5.00
SUNDAY ....2.00 - 5.00
ADMISSION: CHARGE
SHOP. TOILETS.

   ♿ DISABLED ACCESS TO ALL MUSEUM.

   🚶 GROUPS BY APPOINTMENT WITH TALKS.

Known as 'The Queen of the Inland Spas' Harrogate became popular during the Victorian era. The Royal Pump Room was built in 1842 to provide better cover for the rich and fashionable who came to visit the wells and drink the sulphur waters. The Museum charts the history and development of the spa from its humble beginnings to its unrivalled position as a leading European Spa with vivid descriptions of amazing 'cures' and a rare, original bath chair. There is also a collection of ceramics, glass, jewellery, costume, bicycles and toys. The sulphur water can still be tasted.

EDEN CAMP

MALTON
NORTH YORKSHIRE

☎ TELEPHONE: 0653-697 777
OPEN: DAILY ....10.00 - 5.00
        14TH FEBRUARY - 23RD DECEMBER
        LAST ADMISSION 4.00
ADMISSION: CHARGE
TOILETS. REFRESHMENTS. SHOP. JUNIOR ASSAULT
COURSE.

&. DISABLED ACCESS.

In early 1942, a small contingent of army personnel
under the command of a sergeant arrived at Malton. Their
task was to construct a barbed wire enclosure and erect tents
to house the steady flow of enemy prisoners-of-war captured
in North Africa. The site was named Eden Camp and the first
inmates were 250 Italian prisoners. They were put to work
constructing a larger, more permanent camp consisting of 45
huts. Later both Germans and Italians were housed there.
Today a local business man has re-equipped 25 huts to tell
the story of the British people at war. Each hut tells a
different part of the story. In hut 21 the Civil Defence are in
action with members of St. John's Ambulance rescuing a
victim of the Blitz, round the corner the W.V.S. are at work
in a Field Kitchen, and a Red Cross First Aid Post is busily
attending the wounded. This museum will transport you back
to wartime Britain and you will be able to experience the
sights, the sounds, even the smells of those dangerous years.

BECK ISLE MUSEUM OF RURAL LIFE

PICKERING
NORTH YORKSHIRE YO18 8DU

☎ TELEPHONE: 0751-73653
OPEN: MONDAY - SUNDAY ....10.00 - 5.00
        LAST ADMISSION 4.30
        APRIL 1ST - OCTOBER 30TH
ADMISSION: CHARGE

SHOP.

  ♿ DISABLED ACCESS GROUND FLOOR ONLY.

In a handsome stone-built Regency residence near the centre of Pickering, William Marshall, a leading agriculturist of his time, planned England's first Agricultural Institute in the 1800's. To-day the same house contains a collection of bygones relating to the rural crafts and living style of Ryedale. Staffed and operated entirely by volunteers the museum contains a reconstructed cobbler's, village shop, hardware store, wheelwright's shop, blacksmith's, pub and domestic rooms.

Cabinets also display medical and surgical instruments, including a 1930's tonsil guillotine and scalpel, a student's teaching skeleton, pharmacy jars, numerous spectacles and a 19th century electrotherapy machine, jars of magical cures and a book of remedies. Nearby are some veterinary instruments.

ROTUNDA MUSEUM

VERNON ROAD
SCARBOROUGH
NORTH YORKSHIRE

  ✆ TELEPHONE: 0723-374 839

    OPEN: TUESDAY - SUNDAY .... 10.00 - 1.00 & 2.00 - 5.00
               1ST MAY - END SEPTEMBER
               TUESDAY - SATURDAY .... 10.00 - 1.00 & 2.00 - 5.00
               1ST OCTOBER - 30TH APRIL
    ADMISSION: FREE
    SHOP.

  ♿ DISABLED ACCESS - STEPS TO ENTRANCE.

The promotion of sea-water both for drinking and bathing using the 'bathing machines' as a health cure (Scarborough has the first recorded evidence for naked sea-bathing in 1735) made Scarborough a popular town for holidays and health cures in the 18th and 19th centuries.

The museum has a photographic display of the town's rise to fame and much other archival material of prints and paintings. It was still possible to take the waters up to the 1940/50's but today that is no longer available.

THIRSK MUSEUM

16 KIRKGATE
THIRSK
NORTH YORKSHIRE Y07 1JZ

☏ TELEPHONE: 0845-522 755
OPEN: MONDAY - SATURDAY.....................................9.30 - 5.00
         SUNDAY...2.00 - 4.00
         EASTER - END OCTOBER
ADMISSION: CHARGE
SHOP.

♿ DISABLED ACCESS TO GROUND FLOOR ONLY.

Thomas Lord, the founder of Lord's Cricket Ground, was born in 16 Kirkgate in 1755. Now home to a folk museum of the life and work of the people of Thirsk, whose entrance is through the Tourist Information Centre, the museum has a wide range of varied bygones. Cobbler's and blacksmith's tools, Victorian clothing, dolls and games, a reconstructed Victorian kitchen and bedroom. Some pharmaceutical items, belonging to a local chemist, are on display and include a cashier machine, named bottles, pill machine, powder folder and pestle and mortar.

Another local celebrity was 'James Herriot' and a room is devoted to his life as a vet with some of his veterinary equipment.

RYEDALE FOLK MUSEUM

HUTTON-LE-HOLE
YORK
NORTH YORKSHIRE Y06 6UA

☏ TELEPHONE: 07515-367
OPEN: MONDAY - SUNDAY ....10.30 - 5.30
         LAST ADMISSION 4.45
         MID MARCH - END OCTOBER
ADMISSION: CHARGE

SHOP. TOILETS. REFRESHMENTS IN VILLAGE.

  ♿ DISABLED ACCESS TO ALL SITES.

This open-air museum, stretching over a 2.5 acre site in the lovely village of Hutton-le-Hole, was opened in 1964 to house the private collections of Wilfred Crosland, Raymond Hayes and Bertram Frank (the first curator). 13 buildings have been rescued including a cruck cottage, 16th century manor house, helm shed, wagon shed with many farm carts and wagons, crofter's cottage, Edwardian photographic studio, bow-top caravan, blacksmith's forge, and workshops. In these, demonstrations of the ancient crafts can be seen: the tinsmith, shoemaker and cooper. There are also the shops of the cabinet maker, saddler and chemist. The latter has a superb drug run for the dry drugs, a pill-making machine, pestle and mortar, vaccination shield and water filter. The extensive array of bottles contains cobalt blue ones for syrups, green fluted ones for poisons, and large carboys in the window containing only coloured water.

YORK CASTLE MUSEUM

YORK YO1 1RY
NORTH YORKSHIRE

☉ TELEPHONE: 0904-653 611

    OPEN: MONDAY - SATURDAY .... 9.30 - 5.30
              SUNDAY .... 10.00 - 5.30
              APRIL - OCTOBER
              MONDAY - SATURDAY .... 9.30 - 4.00
              SUNDAY .... 10.00 - 4.00
              NOVEMBER - MARCH
    ADMISSION: CHARGE
    TOILETS. REFRESHMENTS. SHOP.

  ♿ DISABLED ACCESS TO GROUND FLOOR (FREE).

  ☏ SCHOOLS BOOKING SERVICE CALL 0904-633 932.

Housed in 18th century prison buildings the Museum was the brainchild of a general practitioner working in North Yorkshire in the 1890's. Dr. Kirk saw a way of life changing and realised the need to collect everyday objects before they were lost forever. Some items he accepted in payment for medical bills, others were gifts or purchases. In 1935 he agreed to give his collection to the City of York and supervised the making of the first displays which opened in 1938. The street and room settings were revolutionary in their design and they brought the past alive by showing how the objects would have been used. The apothecary's shop in Kirkgate commemorates Kirk's home town of Pickering. The contents include glass and Delph jars, leech jars, water filter, phrenologist's head (1855), stomach pump, amputation set, dental instruments, medicine chest, scarifier, cupping set and a stethoscope. Other shops include a printer, optical instrument maker, shoemaker, clock maker, draper, music and accessory shop. Agricultural bygones, a farmhouse kitchen and dairy, domestic bygones and period rooms from a Jacobean dining room to a fifties front room complete this fascinating museum of social history.

South Yorkshire

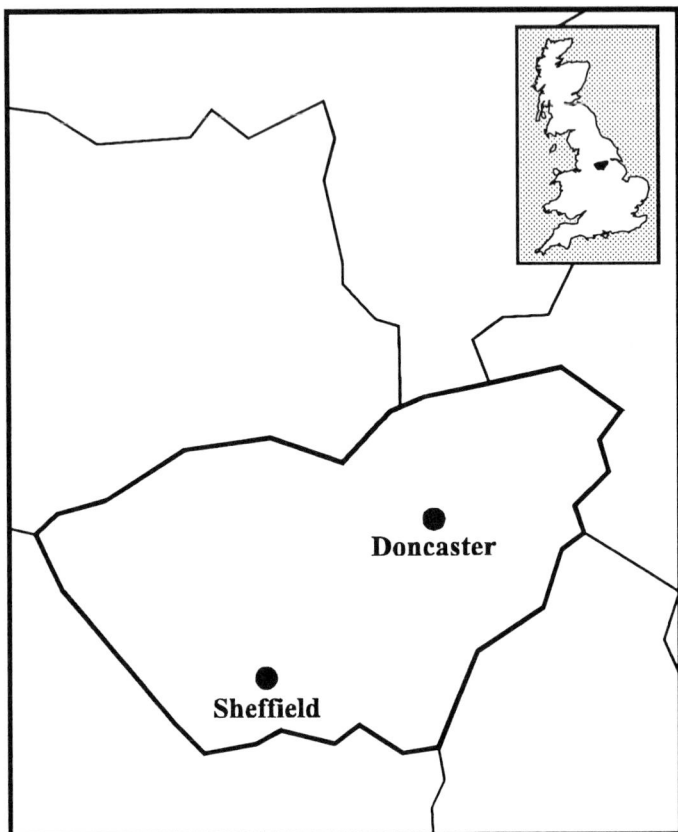

MUSEUM OF SOUTH YORKSHIRE LIFE

CUSWORTH HALL
DONCASTER
SOUTH YORKSHIRE DN5 7TU

TELEPHONE: 0302-782 342
OPEN: MONDAY - FRIDAY .... 10.00 - 5.00
SATURDAY.. 11.00 - 5.00
SUNDAY .... 1.00 - 5.00
EARLY CLOSING DECEMBER/JANUARY 4.00
ADMISSION: FREE
TOILETS. SHOP.

& DISABLED ACCESS TO GROUND FLOOR.

A delightful country house built in the 1740's and set in attractive park land the Hall is now a museum with collections illustrating the way South Yorkshire people have lived, worked and entertained themselves over the past 200 years. The collections include costume, domestic items and kitchen equipment, material on childhood, education, leisure, local transport and industries, crafts and agricultural equipment. One display is a showcase of a chemist's shop window. Reserve collections can be seen by appointment.

KELHAM ISLAND

OFF ALMA STREET
SHEFFIELD
SOUTH YORKSHIRE S3 8RY

☾ TELEPHONE: 0742-722 106
    OPEN: TUESDAY - SATURDAY ....10.00 - 5.00
                  SUNDAY...11.00 - 5.00
    ADMISSION: CHARGE
    SHOP. REFRESHMENTS.
& DISABLED ACCESS.

Sited on an island in the River Don the museum shows Sheffield's industrial heritage in imposing surroundings. The 12,000hp steam engine, which takes 6 people to get it going, runs smoothly for 2 minutes on the hour at 11, 12, 2, 3, and sometimes 4 o'clock. In the transport section is the 1921 Richardson car, the Ner-a Car motor cycle and a silver-plated penny-farthing made for a Russian Tsar. Working at Sheffield's traditional industries are 4 'Little Mesters' - a knife grinder, a cutler making pen and pocket knives, a surgical instrument maker who forges the instruments from steel and a maker of general surgical (mosquito, Spencer Wells and spring forceps) and dental instruments. They are at work most days but especially at week-ends and are very willing to show and share their craftsmanship that has made Sheffield world renowned in this field.

SHEFFIELD CITY MUSEUM

WESTON PARK
SHEFFIELD S10 2TP
SOUTH YORKSHIRE

⊘ TELEPHONE: 0742-768 588
OPEN: TUESDAY - SATURDAY .... 10.00 - 5.00
SUNDAY .... 11.00 - 5.00
ADMISSION: FREE
SHOP. REFRESHMENTS. TOILETS IN ART GALLERY NEXT
DOOR.

& DISABLED ACCESS.

⅄ GUIDED TOURS FOR PRE-BOOKED SCHOOL PARTIES.

Sheffield has a long history in the manufacture of surgical instruments, some of which can be seen in the City Museum, in the often changing displays. In the ceramic gallery are a selection of English delft drug jars (dated 1662). Available by appointment are a late 18th century trepanning set, various folding lancets and an Arnold and Sons instrument catalogue dated January 1885. More instruments, mainly amputation knives and folding lancets are at the Visitor Centre, Globe Works, Penistone Road, Sheffield.

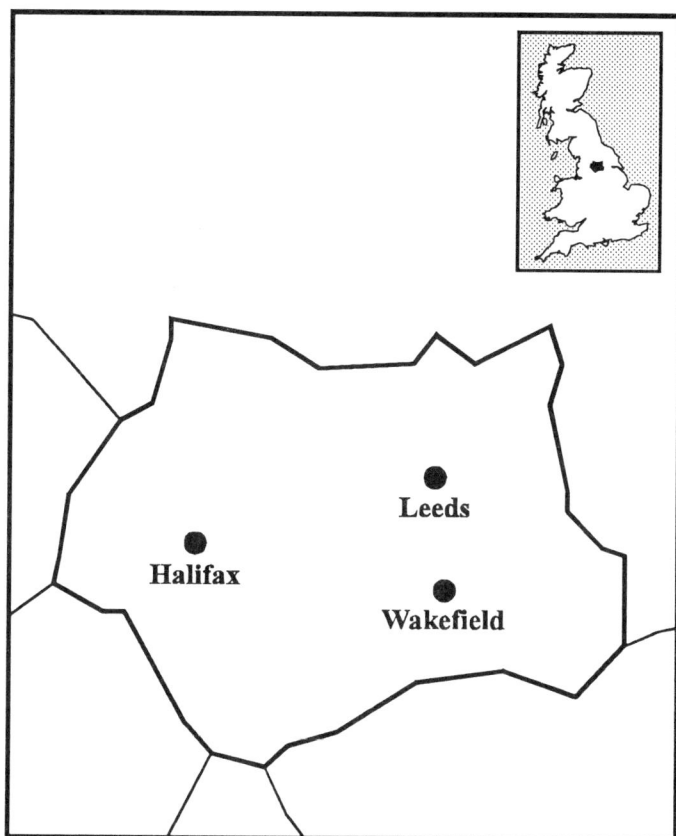

SHIBDEN HALL FOLK MUSEUM

SHIBDEN PARK
HALIFAX
WEST YORKSHIRE HX3 6XG

☎ TELEPHONE: 0422-321 455
     OPEN: MONDAY - SATURDAY.................................10.00 - 6.00
                    SUNDAY..2.00 - 5.00
                    CLOSES 1 HR EARLIER IN OCTOBER, NOVEMBER
                    & MARCH
                    FEBRUARY SUNDAY ONLY ....2.00 - 5.00
     CLOSED: DECEMBER & JANUARY

ADMISSION: CHARGE
SHOP. REFRESHMENTS. TOILETS.

  ♿ DISABLED ACCESS TO GROUND FLOOR ONLY.

  🚶 GUIDED TOURS AVAILABLE.

This 15th century half-timbered house has an atmosphere of being still lived in, with items (from different periods) left about just as they would have been if the person had gone out for a moment. The magnificent 17th century barn houses a collection of horse drawn vehicles, early agricultural implements and a brewhouse. Around the courtyard are craft workshops, an estate worker's cottage, the Crispin Inn and an Apothecary. This has an impressive array of jars and bottles, a pestle and mortar, pill board, and iron clamp for compressing corks to fit the bottle necks, a phrenology head and, in the back area of the shop, a still for the distillation of potions.

ABBEY HOUSE MUSEUM

ABBEY ROAD
KIRKSTALL
LEEDS LS5 3EH
WEST YORKSHIRE

  ☎ TELEPHONE: 0532-755 821
      OPEN: MONDAY - SATURDAY .... 10.00 - 6.00
              SUMMER
              SUNDAY .... 2.00 - 6.00
              WINTER CLOSES ONE HOUR EARLIER
      ADMISSION: CHARGE
      SHOP. TOILETS. CATERING BY PRIOR ARRANGEMENT
      ONLY.

  ♿ DISABLED ACCESS TO GROUND FLOOR.

  🚶 GUIDED TOURS FOR GROUPS.

Once the great Gatehouse of Kirkstall Abbey, whose substantial ruin is across the road, Abbey House after nearly 800 hundred years of continuous occupation, the last 400 hundred as a private home, became a Museum in 1925. The Norman Hall is still intact and now welcomes visitors to explore the life and skills of the people of Leeds at work and play. The Museum possesses a large collection of costumes and accessories, a fascinating toy collection from 1750 to the present day, and an extensive display of domestic appliances and utensils. Three streets of the late 18th and 19th centuries show the workshops and shops typical of the many 'Folds, Courts, Gates and Yards' so common in old Leeds. An ironmonger's, a grocer's, clay-pipe maker's, saddler, blacksmith, weaver, tin-tack maker, wheelwright and joiner together with the chemist's shop can stir the memories. For many years the Castelow family have had their chemist's shop in Woodhouse Lane. The interior fittings date from 1891 and the assorted drug jars and bottles, scales, pill-making equipment, patent medicines, feeding cups, bandages and assorted medicines make a comprehensive display.

THACKRAY MEDICAL MUSEUM

131 BECKETT STREET
LEEDS LS9M 7LP
WEST YORKSHIRE

Ⓓ TELEPHONE: 0532 444343
OPEN: BY APPOINTMENT ONLY

At present this museum is in an interim period and therefore open by appointment only. A completed medical museum showing medicine in the context of everyday living is expected to open in mid-1996 in the magnificently restored old workhouse building.

STEPHEN BEAUMONT MUSEUM

STANLEY ROYD HOSPITAL
ABERFORD ROAD
WAKEFIELD
WEST YORKSHIRE

Ⓓ TELEPHONE: 0924-201 688
OPEN: WEDNESDAYS ONLY.............10.30 - 1.00 & 1.30 - 4.00
(RING FIRST)
OTHER TIMES BY ARRANGEMENT.

ADMISSION: FREE

 ♿   DISABLED ACCESS.

The museum depicts the history of the Stanley Royd Hospital, formerly the 'West Riding Pauper Lunatic Asylum', founded in 1818. The collection includes surgical equipment and instruments, venesection set, leucotomy set and anaesthetic equipment, instruments of restraint, artisans' tools, a padded cell and examples of the skill and artistry of the patients. There is also much archival material of photographs, records, case books, and documents including some Royal signed manuals of Kings George IV, William IV and Queen Victoria.

The hospital is due to close by the Spring of 1995 so the future of the museum is far from certain.

SCOTLAND

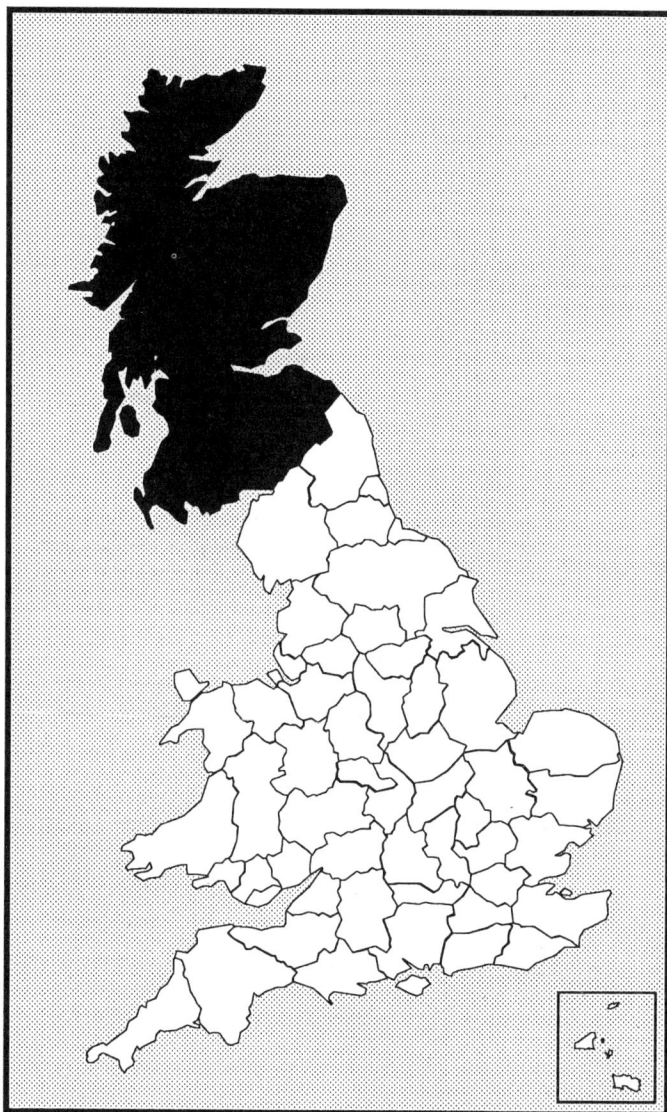

Dumfries & Galloway

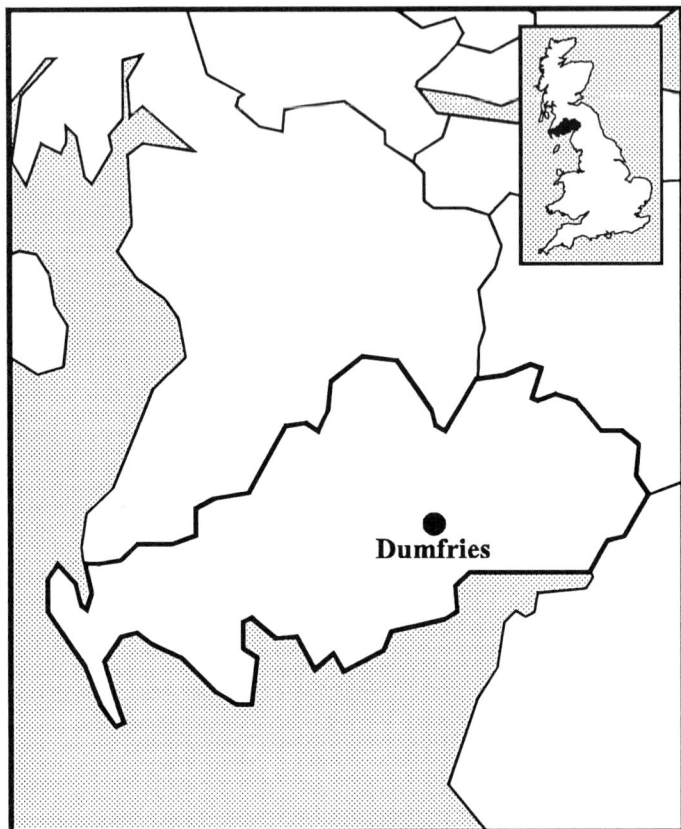

DUMFRIES MUSEUM

THE OBSERVATORY
DUMFRIES
DUMFRIES AND GALLOWAY DG2 7SW

☎ TELEPHONE: 0387-53374
OPEN: MONDAY - SATURDAY .... 10.00 - 1.00 & 2.00 - 5.00
              SUNDAY .... 2.00 - 5.00
CLOSED SUNDAY & MONDAY .... OCTOBER - MARCH
ADMISSION: FREE
CAMERA OBSCURA
CLOSED OCTOBER - MARCH

ADMISSION:
>   MUSEUM, FREE
>   CAMERA OBSCURA, CHARGE
> SHOP. REFRESHMENTS AT ROBERT BURNS CENTRE
> 100 YARDS, TO END SEPTEMBER.

  ♿   DISABLED ACCESS WITH LIFT TO FIRST FLOOR.

Situated in the 18th century windmill tower on top of Corbelly Hill is the local museum which was started over 150 years ago. The Camera Obscura is to be found on the top floor of the windmill when it was converted into an observatory in 1836. The museum has prehistoric fossil foot-prints, early tools and weapons, stone carvings by Scotland's first Christians, rich and varied artefacts from the locality and everyday items of the Victorian farm, workshop and home.

There is an exhibition on medicine which deals with local medical practice from the 1600's, covering the plague, cholera, herbal medicines, the development of surgery, the establishment of a local hospital and the first use of anaesthetic ether. Objects on display include mortars and pestles, a leech jar, medical receipt book, herbal and pharmacopoeia, issue peas, medical instruments of the 1840's and surgical instruments of the 1940's, a collection of patent medicines, an apothecary's cabinet and travelling medicine boxes.

OLD BRIDGE HOUSE MUSEUM

> MILL ROAD
> DUMFRIES
> DUMFRIES AND GALLOWAY DG2 7BE

① TELEPHONE: 0387-56904
>   OPEN: MONDAY - SATURDAY........... 10.00 - 1.00 & 2.00 - 5.00
>   SUNDAY...2.00 - 5.00
>   APRIL - SEPTEMBER
> ADMISSION: FREE
> SHOP. REFRESHMENTS AND TOILETS AT ROBERT BURNS
> CENTRE 200 YDS.

  ♿   NO DISABLED ACCESS.

Built in 1660 into the fabric of the bridge, Dumfries's oldest house is now a museum of everyday life in the town. It contains several period rooms showing kitchens of 1850 and 1900, Victorian childhood and an early dentist's surgery. This shows the instruments, drills, chair and equipment used by the dentist at the beginning of this century.

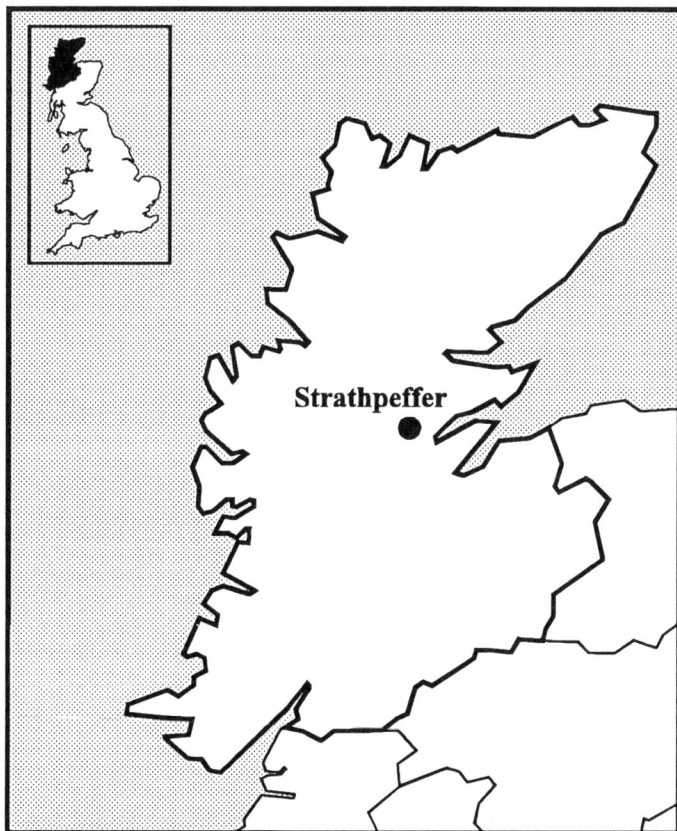

WATER SAMPLING PAVILION

THE SQUARE
STRATHPEFFER SPA
HIGHLAND
SCOTLAND

TELEPHONE: 0997 421 415
OPEN: MONDAY - SUNDAY ....9.00 - 6.00
             EASTER - OCTOBER
ADMISSION: FREE
SHOP. TOURIST INFORMATION CENTRE.

The hideaway village of Strathpeffer is Britain's most northerly spa and was very popular with the Victorians, tucked away amongst the grandeur of Scotland's glens and lochs. Created as a holiday resort much of the impressive Victorian architecture remains today. The sulphur waters can be tasted at the Pavilion and the newly restored Pump Room during the summer months.

Lothian

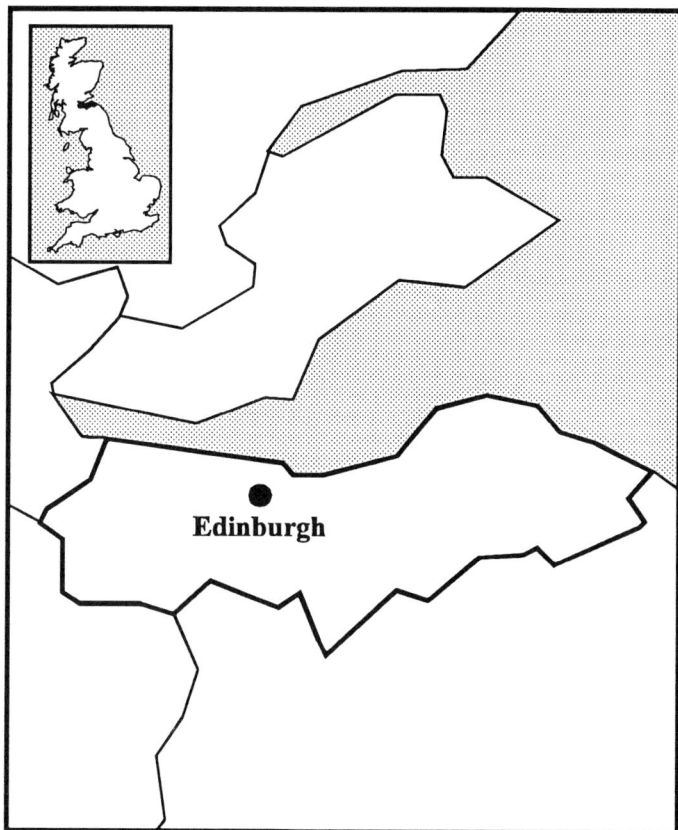

ROYAL MUSEUM OF SCOTLAND

CHAMBERS STREET
EDINBURGH EH1 1JF
SCOTLAND

TELEPHONE: 031-225 7534
OPEN: MONDAY - SATURDAY ....10.00 - 5.00
            SUNDAY ....2.00 - 5.00
ADMISSION: FREE
LIBRARY OPEN BY APPOINTMENT
SHOP. REFRESHMENTS. TOILETS. EXTENSIVE RANGE OF
TALKS, LECTURES ACTIVITIES, FIELD TRIPS AND FILMS.

 ♿   DISABLED ACCESS.

In one of Edinburgh's finest Victorian buildings of glass and iron begun in 1860 as a museum of science and art, the Royal Museum is now part of the National Museums of Scotland. They hold international and Scottish material in geology and natural history, archaeology and ethnography, the decorative arts and science and technology.

In the latter department are a range of medico-scientific instruments from early Florentine thermometers; microscopes from France, Germany and London; applications for optical instruments in the late 19th century; electrical equipment; information on Monro *primus* (1697-1767) and the case book of the private practice of Andrew Sinclair (1697-1760). Also applications of the microscope in the late 19th century when it was beginning to be used in the clinical investigation of disease with a microscope slide preparation kit of R.J. Beck of London of 1870 and a Zeiss instrument of 1900.

THE SIR JULES THORN HISTORICAL MUSEUM

      THE ROYAL COLLEGE OF SURGEONS
      NICHOLSON STREET
      EDINBURGH EH8 9DW
      LOTHIAN
      SCOTLAND

 ☎   TELEPHONE: 031-556 6206
      OPEN: MONDAY - FRIDAY ....2.00 - 4.00
      ADMISSION: FREE
      PLAYFAIR MUSEUM OF PATHOLOGY OPEN BY
      APPOINTMENT ONLY.
      MENZIES CAMPBELL DENTAL COLLECTION OPEN BY
      APPOINTMENT ONLY (END 1993.)
      TOILET.
 ♿   NO DISABLED ACCESS.

This new museum tells the history of the surgeons and anatomists who earned Edinburgh its international fame as a centre of medical teaching. It leads from the founding of the College in 1505 to the present day.

There is a facsimile Peter Lowe's book 'Whole Course of Chirurgerie', the first textbook of surgery to be written in English, dedicated by the Glasgow surgeon to Gilbert Primrose of Edinburgh. Panels describe the early meeting places of the surgeons and apothecaries and there is a reconstructed 18th century apothecary's shop and a catalogue of plants from the Edinburgh Physic Garden of 1683. Archibald Pitcairn was a surgeon in 1703/4 and his portrait hangs together with 2 early anatomical preparations showing the blood vessels of the hand and foot. By the Monro family connection, the Royal Infirmary was founded in 1729 on the instigation of Alexander, the son, whilst the father was influential in establishing a proper medical school at the University by 1720. Edinburgh's influence on early American medicine is illustrated and it was graduates from the City who established the first medical school at Philadelphia in 1765. Robert Knox, the anatomist and first Conservator of the Museum is shown working in his study.

Military surgery is displayed with Bell's book on wounds, a bullet extractor and a skeleton with gunshot wounds. Burke and Hare, the infamous 'body-snatchers', have a descriptive case as do Robert Liston and James Syme, two eminent 19th century surgeons. Instruments include Liston's amputation knives, Simpson's obstetric forceps and examples of the different techniques and pins used by Lister when treating fractures. A 19th century dental surgery is reconstructed.

The upper gallery is devoted to some aspects of current surgical practice in various specialities including a paediatric operating theatre.

Strathclyde

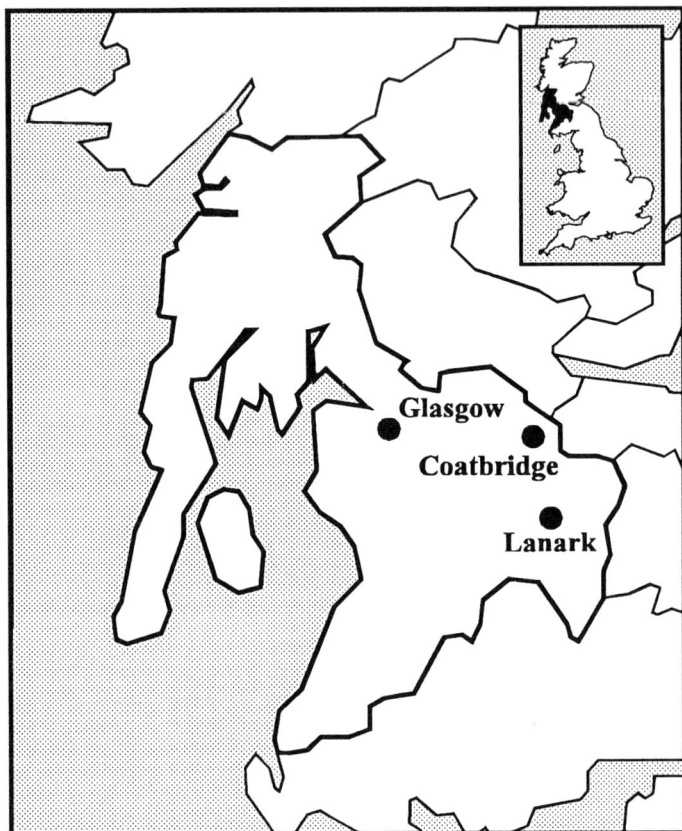

SUMMERLEE HERITAGE TRUST

WEST CANAL STREET
COATBRIDGE
STRATHCLYDE ML5 1QD
SCOTLAND

☎ TELEPHONE: 0236-431 261
OPEN: DAILY .... 10.00 - 5.00
            EXCEPT CHRISTMAS/NEW YEAR PERIOD
ADMISSION: FREE
TOILETS. REFRESHMENTS. SHOP. CANALSIDE PICNIC AND
PLAY AREA.

  ♿ DISABLED ACCESS.

150 years ago Summerlee Ironworks were at the hub of the Industrial revolution when coal and iron brought prosperity to Scotland's Iron Burgh. 50 years ago the works became derelict and forgotten but today the site preserves and interprets the history of the former iron, steel and engineering industries and the communities that depended upon them for a living. The massive exhibition hall features the clatter of belt-driven machinery and the hiss of gas engines and, in daily operation, are a spade forge, brass finishers shop and Victorian trade exhibition. The social gallery has some items on midwifery from the 1930-1950's including three nurses' bags, forceps, syringes, dressings, obstetric stethoscope, 'Durban' breast reliever and several books, one dated 1925 'C.M.B. Examination Questions'. Also an ambulance and mortuary trolley, three stretchers, a 'Sparklets' resuscitator and several rows of bottles and shelving from a local chemist. Outside visitors may ride on Scotland's only working electric tramway, in operation daily, and see the historic steam engines in action regularly.

DEPARTMENT OF ANATOMY, GLASGOW UNIVERSITY

UNIVERSITY OF GLASGOW
UNIVERSITY AVENUE
GLASGOW G12 8QQ
STRATHCLYDE
SCOTLAND

  ☎ TELEPHONE: 041-339 8855 EXT. 4296
     OPEN: BY APPOINTMENT ONLY
  ♿ DISABLED ACCESS TO GROUND FLOOR ONLY.

This purpose-built galleried museum of 1870 contains not only the anatomical and pathological specimens prepared by William Hunter himself but those of later anatomists and contemporary teaching aids. Hunter's own specimens are principally in the upper gallery and include plaster casts of the abdomen in pregnancy made from his original dissections. Most of his work on the uterus and specimens of the gravid uterus and abnormal foetuses are also upstairs. A case showing his life and work is on the ground floor.

Many of his books and manuscripts are held by the Hunterian Museum and the University Library.

HUNTERIAN MUSEUM

UNIVERSITY AVENUE
UNIVERSITY OF GLASGOW
GLASGOW
STRATHCLYDE
SCOTLAND G12 8QQ

℺ TELEPHONE: 041 330 4221
OPEN: MONDAY - SATURDAY .... 9.30 - 5.00
ADMISSION: FREE
SHOP. COFFEE SHOP. VISITOR CENTRE IN MAIN BUILDING
WITH SNACKS & TOILETS.

♿ DISABLED ACCESS BY PRIOR APPOINTMENT.

🚶 GROUPS BY APPOINTMENT.

William Hunter was born at Long Calderwood Farm, East Kilbride, near Glasgow in 1718. At the age of 13 he became a student in the Faculty of Arts at Glasgow University where he studied for 5 years. Although destined for the Church, on the advice of his father, Hunter met Dr. Cullen, a doctor practising at Hamilton, and decided to devote himself to the profession of physic. He studied medicine at Edinburgh and London and received his degree of Doctor of Medicine from Glasgow University in 1750. His reputation as a surgeon, anatomist and obstetrician grew quickly especially after he was called to attend Queen Charlotte's first confinement in 1764. In 1770 he moved into a purpose built house in Great Windmill Street, London with a dissecting-room, lecture theatre, and museum hall. His museum contained not only his pathology specimens but objects of archaeology, natural history, geology, mineralogy and an extensive coin collection. At his death in 1783 his collection and paintings, prints, books and manuscripts and substantial funding to enable the building of a suitable museum were bequeathed to Glasgow University.

Housed in the University buildings of 1870 some of his instruments, specimens and the 'Gravid Uterus' of 1774 are on display in the permanent exhibition 'An Overflowing Fountain' which tells the story of the University's growth and achievements. Other items include a microscope made by John Marshall in 1680, Ayscough's Apparatus of 1726, James Watt's workshop, tools and a model of the Newcomen Engine in 1756, a microscope of Lister's father, a model of an operating table used by Lister and his surgical instruments and spray, phials of urine (reported to be his own) and a sterilisation unit. An early 1900's electric shock machine, ophthalmascope and instrument case and a display of Glasgow's first medical school for women established in 1890 by Mrs. Galloway.

A new exhibition 'Earth Life' will trace the evolution of the solar system, the rise of life on Earth and the many different ways humans have lived on this planet, including a fine collection of Roman material.

PEOPLE'S PALACE

GLASGOW GREEN
GLASGOW
STRATHCLYDE
SCOTLAND

ⓓ TELEPHONE: 041-554 0223
OPEN: MONDAY - SATURDAY................................10.00 - 5.00
SUNDAY..11.00 - 5.00
ADMISSION: FREE
SHOP. REFRESHMENTS. TOILETS.

 ♿ DISABLED ACCESS.

 🕴 GROUPS BY APPOINTMENT.

Built in 1888 as a multi-purpose cultural centre for the people living in Glasgow's eastern side, the museum with a large iron and glass 'conservatory' has been used as a music and concert hall and winter garden. To-day is shows the history of Glasgow with items related to trade and industry, unions and the labour movement, women's suffrage, entertainment and sport. A pharmacy shop front from the early 1900's displays the coloured glass medicine bottles, tins, pots and jars of proprietary and patent medicines, a china nasal douche labelled 'iglodine', a carbolic spray, Boots improved enema syringes, a magneto electro machine for nervous and other diseases, Dr. Macaura's patent blood circulator, a urine testing box, pill rolling and suppository making equipment, electrodes for giving galvanic current to stimulate muscles, obstetric forceps as used in the 1930's and a pharmaceutical cabinet from the Forresthall Hospital.

THE DAVID LIVINGSTONE CENTRE

STATION ROAD
BLANTYRE
GLASGOW G72 9BT
STRATHCLYDE
SCOTLAND

☎ TELEPHONE: 0698-823 140
OPEN: MONDAY - SATURDAY .... 10.00 - 6.00
SUNDAY .... 2.00 - 6.00
LAST ENTRY TO MUSEUM 5.15
ADMISSION: CHARGE
LIBRARY: OPEN BY APPOINTMENT TO SERIOUS
RESEARCHERS.
SHOP. REFRESHMENTS. TOILETS. PARK. CHILDREN'S
ADVENTURE PLAYGROUND.

 ♿ DISABLED ACCESS TO GROUND FLOOR AND AFRICAN
PAVILION BY ARRANGEMENT.

 👫 PARTIES BY ARRANGEMENT.

The 18th century tenement house, which once housed 24 families, is where David Livingstone was born in 1813 and lived in one room on the top floor landing with his parents and sister. The building is now a museum with the Livingstone's room re-created with box-beds, dresser, fire, rag rug, and spinning wheel. The young Livingstone aged 10 worked for 14 hours a day in the local cotton mill, learning Latin while he worked. At 23 he studied theology, Greek and medicine at Anderson's College in Glasgow and in 1837 applied to work for the London Missionary Society. In 1839 he came to London to complete his medical studies at

Charing Cross Hospital and Moorfields, qualifying in Glasgow in 1840.

Prevented by war from working in China, he was attracted to Africa by Dr. Moffat. He left on 8th December 1840 and went straight to the mission station in Bechuanaland, later marrying Moffat's daughter Mary. Besides teaching and ministering for many years Livingstone made numerous journeys of exploration in Africa and, finally feared lost or dead, he had his famous meeting with Stanley in 1871 at Ujiji. Two years later he died and his body was brought back to lie in Westminster Abbey.

The museum traces his work in Africa and has many of his personal items on display including his watch, sextant, boxed compass, consul uniform and boots, his pocket surgical instruments, microscope, metal medicine case, card of surgical needles, amputation kit and some of his notebooks and letters. One letter is from his daughter to Hans Christian Anderson. The African Pavilion has many items for sale from Zambia and a colourful craft exhibition. The Blantyre story tells about the surrounding area and small exhibitions are mounted frequently.

NEW LANARK CONSERVATION VILLAGE

NEW LANARK MILLS
LANARK
STRATHCLYDE ML11 9DB

① TELEPHONE: 0555-61345
OPEN: DAILY ....11.00 - 5.00
          GUIDED TOURS FROM................................10.15 - 3.30
ADMISSION: CHARGE
TOILETS. REFRESHMENTS. SHOP. PICNIC AREA.
ADVENTURE PLAYGROUND. WALKS IN FALL OF CLYDE
NATURE RESERVE.

♿ DISABLED ACCESS TO VISITOR CENTRE (INC. MILL THREE)

In 1784 David Dale brought Richard Arkwright, the inventor of the water frame, to the Falls of Clyde, a deep marshy valley far from Glasgow and reached by bad roads. The plentiful supply of cheap energy encouraged Dale to establish cotton spinning mills at Lanark. Robert Owen, the manager in the early 1800's, introduced a series of social and educational reforms designed to improve the quality of life for his workforce. These included phasing out the use of child labour and establishing progressive schools, including the world's first nursery school. The village store was run for the benefit of the community and is regarded as the cradle of the co-operative movement. He instituted free medical care for the workers and surgeons were employed to care for the health of the villagers, mill workers and 'bug hunters', a type of early health visitor scheme. Health and hygiene were considered very important by Owen and, although no remnants of the actual premises of the surgeries survive, documentary evidence does exist and the staff at the Mills are well informed on Owen's new ideas. The 'Annie McLeod Experience' offers a glimpse of life in New Lanark in 1820 as the spirit of 10-year-old Annie shows you her living conditions and explains how Owen's reforming ideas affected the lives of ordinary people.

Tayside

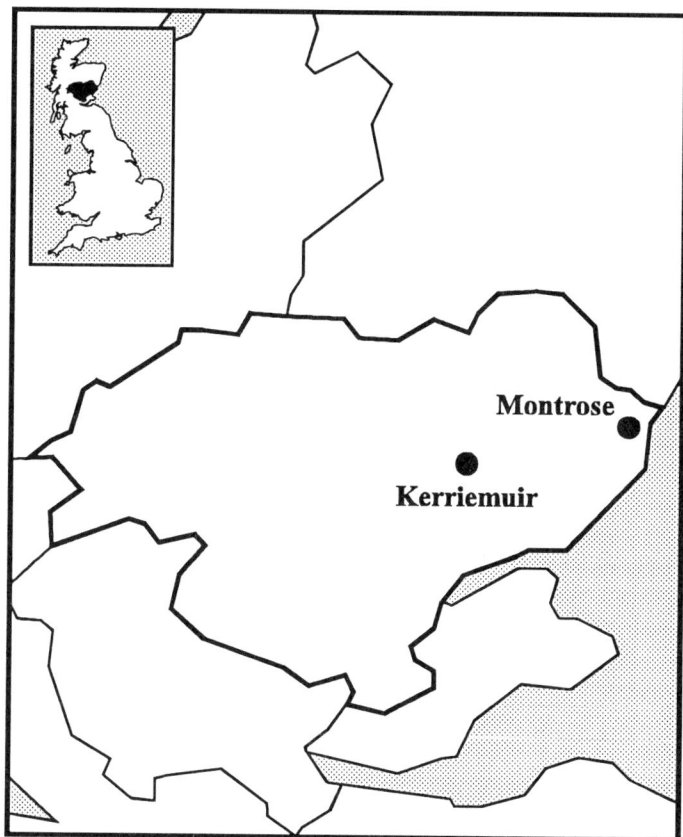

BARRIE'S BIRTHPLACE

9 BRECHIN ROAD
KIRRIEMUIR
ANGUS
TAYSIDE DD8 4BX
SCOTLAND

☏ TELEPHONE: 0575-72646
OPEN: MONDAY - SATURDAY.................................11.00 - 5.30
               SUNDAY...2.00 - 5.30
               LAST ADMISSION 5.00
               1ST MAY - 30TH SEPTEMBER & EASTER WEEKEND

ADMISSION: CHARGE
SHOP. REFRESHMENTS.
  ♿   DISABLED ACCESS TO GROUND FLOOR ONLY.

J.M. Barrie, author and playwright, was born here in 1860. The upper floors are furnished as they may have been when Barrie lived here. The adjacent house, No. 11, holds a new exhibition - The Genius of J.M. Barrie - about his literary and theatrical works and contains some of his original manuscripts. The outside wash-house is said to have been his first theatre and the inspiration for the Wendy house in Peter Pan. In 1929 Barrie made a gift of the copyright of Peter Pan to The Hospital for Sick Children at Great Ormond Street, London. This much loved play whether performed on stage, television or in films, and the further book reprints, have given enormous financial support to the hospital. The latest film 'Hook' in 1992 has already raised £200,000 from the premiere alone. Nearby is a small cottage to rent; details from the Scottish National Trust.

SUNNYSIDE ROYAL HOSPITAL

MONTROSE
TAYSIDE DD10 9JP
SCOTLAND

☎ TELEPHONE: 067483-361
OPEN: WEDNESDAY..2.00 - 3.30
             EASTER - NOVEMBER
ADMISSION: FREE
REFRESHMENTS.

The Montrose Lunatic Asylum, Infirmary and Dispensary, the first of its kind in Scotland, came into being in 1781, largely due to the efforts of one remarkable woman, Mrs. Susan Carnegie of Charlton. The first lunatic was admitted on 6th May 1782. After several moves the Asylum came to its present site in 1858 and many of the original minutes, admission forms, salary charts and store accounts still exist. During the second world war in 1940 five high explosive bombs fell on the hospital and the first George Medal in Scotland was awarded to a nurse for her devotion to duty during the raid. To-day the hospital, with four hundred in-patients, has a rehabilitation unit, 'half way houses' and a day hospital. The museum has a wide range of exhibits including a straight jacket, replicas of nursing uniforms worn in the 1890's and reproductions of photographic archives (1890's to just after the great war). A replica of the Tolbooth (where lunatics were imprisoned in the 18th century along with criminals), samples of creative work done by the patients 50 years ago and samples of two sets of cutlery which were used by the pauper and the rich patients respectively can be seen.

WALES

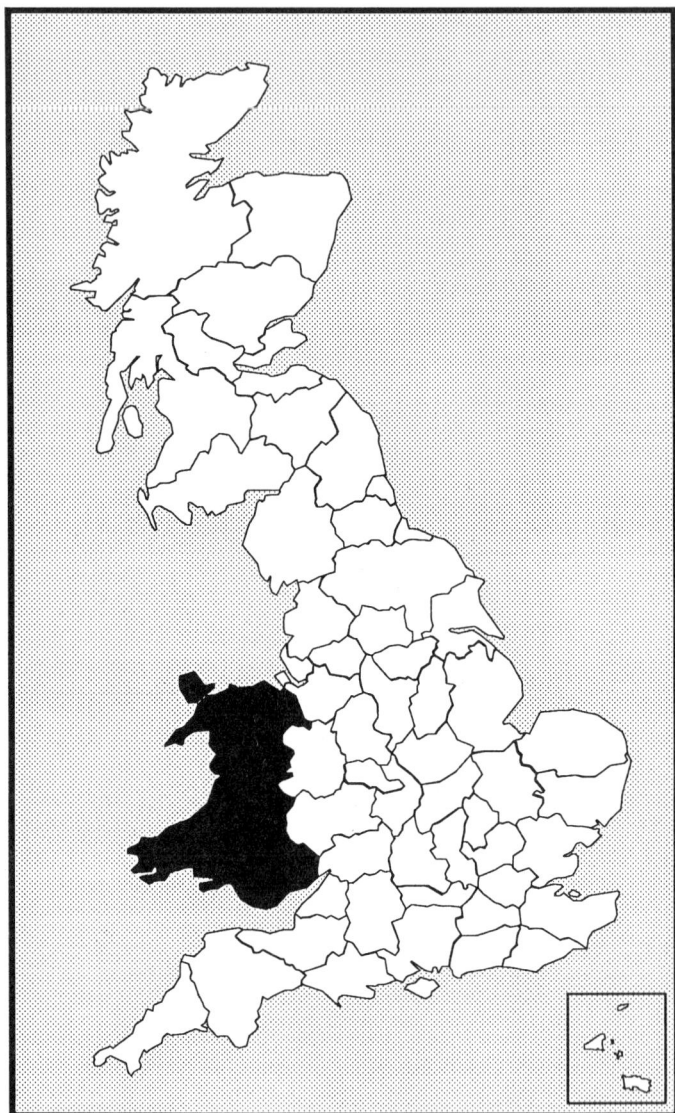

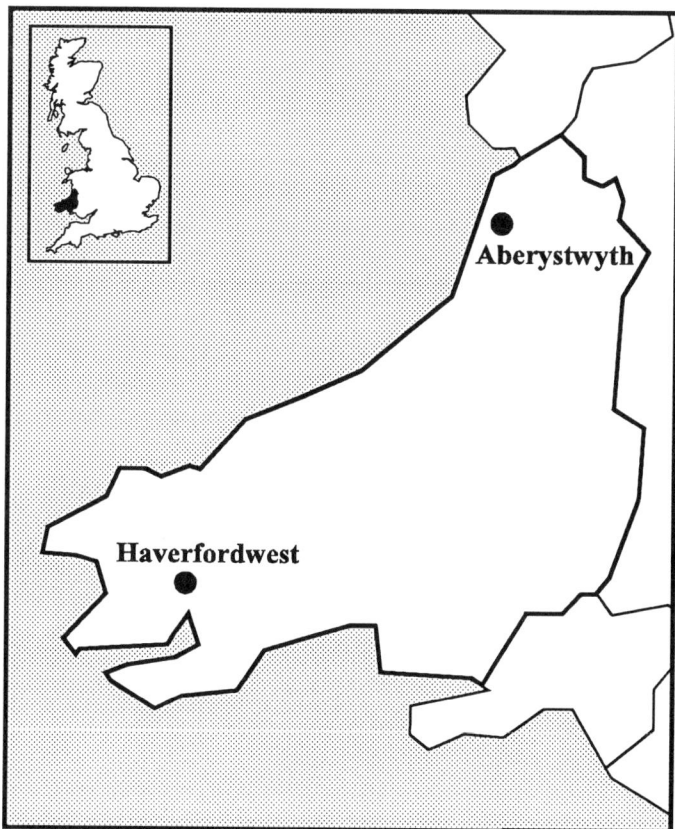

CEREDIGION MUSEUM

COLISEUM
TERRACE ROAD
ABERYSTWYTH
DYFED SY23 2AQ

① TELEPHONE: 0970-617 911
   OPEN: MONDAY - SATURDAY.................................10.00 - 5.00
             SUNDAY DURING SCHOOL HOLIDAYS.
   ADMISSION: CHARGE
   SHOP. TOILETS. REFRESHMENTS NEARBY.

♿ DISABLED ACCESS.

The museum is housed in an Edwardian Music Hall Theatre and displays the local industries, a folk collection, reconstructed cottage interior, domestic bygones, clocks, slate enamelling and a dentist's surgery. The majority of the items came from Mr D.S. Turner in Aberystwyth who retired in 1982, but much of the material was used by his predecessors Mr. D. Dunlop Reid and Mr. Oswald Lloyd. It includes the dentist's chair, instrument tray and burrs, a foot bellows used to operate an air-gas blow pipe to cast gold inlays and drill hand piece date from the 1920/30's. Other items are clamps, polishing strips, pliers, scalpels, syringes, sprays, colour guide books, false teeth and a foot-operated drill.

SCOLTON MANOR MUSEUM

SPITTAL
NEAR HAVERFORDWEST
DYFED

☎ TELEPHONE: 0437-731 328
OPEN: TUESDAY - SUNDAY .... 10.00 - 4.30
ADMISSION: CHARGE
SHOP. REFRESHMENTS. TOILETS. COUNTRY PARK OPEN
ALL YEAR (EXCEPT MONDAY).

♿ DISABLED ACCESS TO GROUND FLOOR.

Set in 60 acres of country park land the Victorian Manor House is the home to the museum of the history and development of Pembrokeshire. The house is being re-furbished in 1992 but the large exhibition hall is open and displays aspects of medieval life, farming and dairy engineering and the county's railways. Some medical items can be seen by appointment such as nursing equipment from a local nurse in Fishguard, 1900 - 1901 uniforms, medicines, tools, implements, bed pans, a tin bath for infants and photographs but a chemist's shop is not yet on display.

Gwent

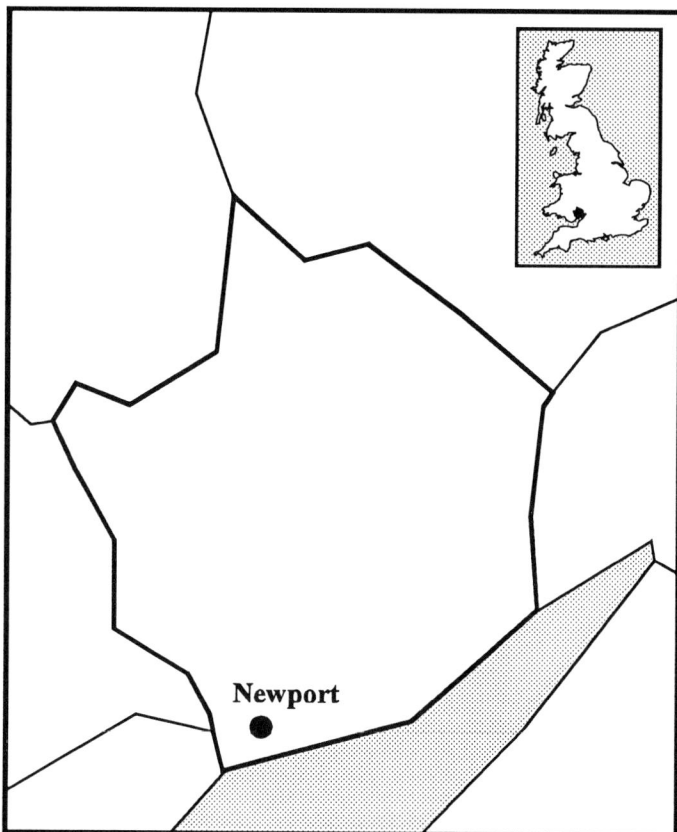

NEWPORT MUSEUM & ART GALLERY

JOHN FROST SQUARE
NEWPORT
GWENT NP9 1HZ

☎ TELEPHONE: 0633-840 064
OPEN: MONDAY - THURSDAY ....9.30 - 5.00
               FRIDAY...9.30 - 4.30
               SATURDAY...9.30 - 4.00
ADMISSION: FREE
SHOP.

♿ DISABLED ACCESS TO FIRST & THIRD FLOORS.

This purpose built modern building overlooks John Frost Square, named after the local tailor, draper and mayor who was sentenced to be hanged, drawn and quartered for leading a Chartist riot in 1839. Instead he was transported for 14 years to Tasmania. The museum has a fascinating archaeology department including material which has been excavated from nearby Caerwent. Amongst these finds are 4 Romano-British medical instruments: the uvula forceps or staphylagra used for the amputation of the uvula and removal of haemorrhoids; a very slender double-ended copper alloy probe with a small olivary terminal at each end; a 'double olive' or dipyrene used for probing a fistulae or possibly removing nasal polyps; a spatula probe used in the preparation and application of medicaments and as a tongue depressor, cautery and blunt dissector. There are other displays on natural science, the domestic and working life of people in and around Gwent and regular exhibitions and lectures.

Gwynedd

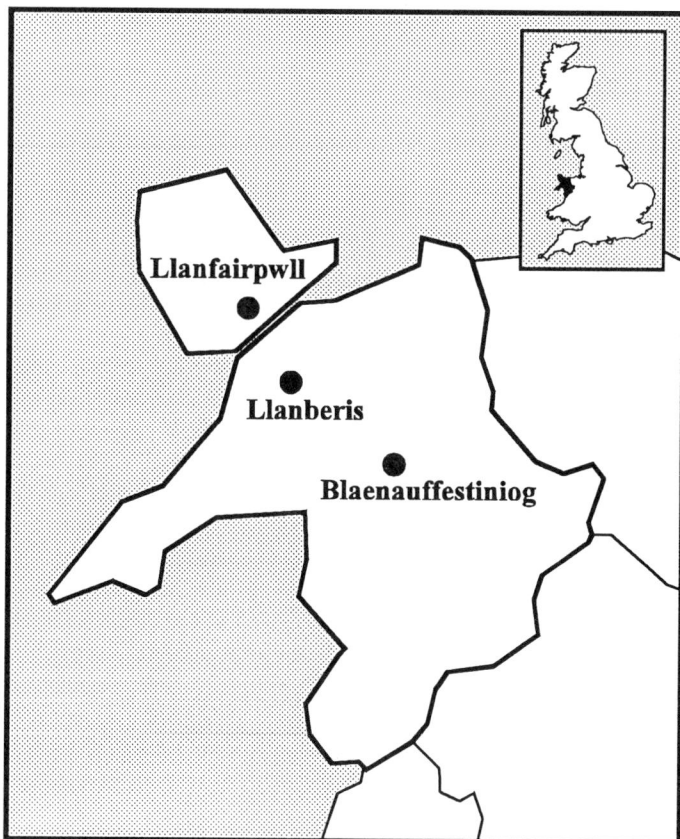

LLECHWEDD SLATE CAVERNS

BLAENAUFFESTINIOG
GWYNEDD LL41 3NB

TELEPHONE: 0766-30306
OPEN: MONDAY - SUNDAY ....10.00 - 5.15
              SITE CLOSES..6.00
              MARCH - SEPTEMBER

              ....10.00 - 4.15
              OCTOBER - FEBRUARY
ADMISSION: CHARGE

SHOP. REFRESHMENTS. TOILETS. RESTAURANT BOOKINGS
ON 0766-830 523.

 ♿ DISABLED ACCESS TO VILLAGE.

In 1972 a half-mile section of the Victorian tramway
through Llechwedd slate caverns was opened to the public.
Today visitors can board a special train to descend on
Britain's steepest passenger incline railway to visit the
caverns, passages and underground lakes that were the
Victorian slate miners' work place. The Miner's Tramway is
a guided tour of the original miner's route of 1846, through a
network of impressive caverns and tableaux. The Victorian
village has a pub, shops, lock-up, harpist cottage and smithy.
In store is the pharmacy of Lloyd Jones, of Blaenauffestiniog
dating from the early part of this century. It is hoped to put
these items on display when space is available.

DINORWIG QUARRY HOSPITAL

PARC PADARN
LLANBERIS
GWYNEDD

☎️ TELEPHONE: 0286-870 892
    OPEN: MONDAY - SUNDAY .... 10.00 - 4.45
             FROM WHIT WEEKEND - END SEPTEMBER
             ALSO EASTER WEEK
    ADMISSION: CHARGE
    SHOP. REFRESHMENTS. TOILETS.

 ♿ DISABLED ACCESS TO GROUND FLOOR, CAN BE DRIVEN TO
FRONT DOOR.

The hospital was built around 1860 overlooking Llyn
Padarn, and officially opened in 1876 by the owner of the
Dinorwig Quarries, Mr. Thomas Assheton-Smith. It was
considered a good policy to maintain a hospital on the site to
treat the fearsome injuries sustained by the slate quarry
workers. Originally there were 20 different rooms, including
a kitchen, a laundry and staff bedrooms. Today the Sister's
room is used for display and an information point, the
Operating Room has the original table, and instruments and
hot and cold running water at the surgeon's sink with pedals

so the taps could be turned off by foot. Thomas splints, a 'Lister Spray', the examination couch totally covered with a fitted 'hot water bottle' for the rapid warming of chilled patients, and a chair made by the quarry workers with an adjustable head-rest for the treatment of eye injuries creates an authentic picture of a nineteenth century emergency hospital. The first X-ray unit in North Wales was used here and the Jackson focus tables from the 1898 machine can be seen. A small ward with 3 iron beds, complete with bed cradles, 'monkey poles', bed pans, tin urinals , a commode and a bed side table which could quickly convert into a seat for a visitor, have been carefully re-created. Charts of accidents at work and fatal accidents are on display but further history of the site, records and documentation are held at Gwynedd Archives Service, Victoria Dock, Caernarfon, Gwynedd LL5 1SH.

PLAS NEWYDD

> LLANFAIRPWLL
> ANGLESEY
> GWYNEDD LL61 6EQ

Ⓣ TELEPHONE: 0248-714 795
OPEN: MONDAY - FRIDAY & SUNDAY.....................12.00 - 5.00
GARDENS..11.00 - 5.00
JULY & AUGUST
1ST APRIL - END SEPTEMBER
FRIDAY & SUNDAY ONLY ....12.00 - 5.00
2ND OCTOBER -1ST NOVEMBER
LAST ADMISSION 4.30
ADMISSION: CHARGE, NATIONAL TRUST
SHOP. REFRESHMENTS. TOILETS.

♿ DISABLED ACCESS TO GROUND FLOOR. SPECIAL PARKING. PLEASE RING.

An 18th century gothic house by James Wyatt is set in beautiful park land over looking the Menai Strait. The gardens include a special Spring garden and children's playground. In the house is Rex Whistler's largest mural and a military museum with relics from the 1st Marquess of Anglesey and the battle of Waterloo. The Marquess led a charge of the Household Cavalry at Waterloo and was badly wounded in the right knee by grapeshot later in battle. The injured leg was amputated the following day, he survived and some years later designed for himself an artificial limb; the first to have a moveable knee joint. The 'Anglesey Leg' has been used as a pattern by the artificial limb makers at the Roehampton centre since World War II.

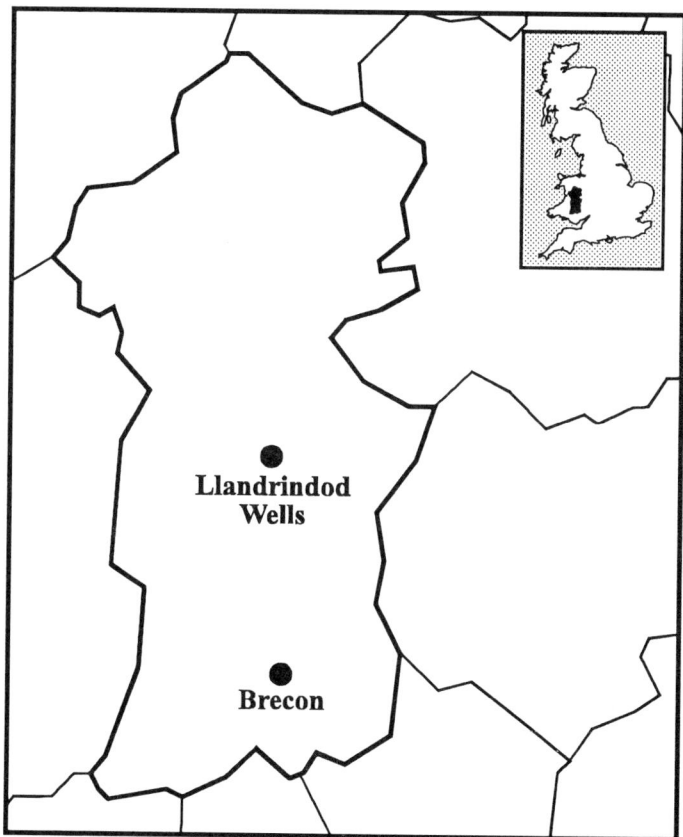

THE HOWELL HARRIS MUSEUM

COLEG TREFECA
ABERHONDDU
BRECKON
POWYS LD3 OPP

TELEPHONE: 0874-711 423
OPEN: MONDAY - SATURDAY...................................9.00 - 6.00
SUMMER
EARLIER CLOSING IN WINTER
ADMISSION: FREE

Trefeca was the birthplace of Howell Harris (1714-1773), the Methodist reformer, where he founded the unique religious-industrial community (1736) which played a significant part in the religious and social history of 18th century Wales. The building stands in 5 acres of peaceful park land and is the Laity Training Centre of the Presbyterian Church of Wales. It is also available for Church groups and other organisations who wish to arrange residential or day conferences. The museum has Harris's portable field pulpit, the turret clock which was added to the clock tower in 1754, household furniture, Harris's swords and guns, a selection of photographs and religious books from the Trevecka Press published between 1770 and 1805, and the telescope which Harris brought in 1761 to record the Transit of Venus over the Sun. His electrifying machine, purchased in 1763, followed the recommendations of John Wesley in his 'Primitive Physick', that it was useful for curing as many as 45 ailments including baldness, blindness, deafness, gout, lunacy, old age and toothache, can be seen.

LLANDRINDOD MUSEUM

TEMPLE STREET
LLANDRINDOD WELLS
POWYS

✆ TELEPHONE: 0597-824 513
OPEN: MONDAY - SUNDAY .... 10.00 - 1.00 & 2.00 - 5.00
              APRIL - SEPTEMBER
CLOSED: SATURDAY AFTERNOONS & SUNDAY
              OCTOBER - APRIL
ADMISSION: FREE
SHOP.

This graceful town set in outstanding scenery was a popular spa during the Victorian and Edwardian eras. The spacious buildings and wide streets set on the shores of a lake still provide a place of relaxation and beauty. The restored Pump Room at the Rock Park serves the famous waters and the museum has a permanent display on the theme of 'Llandrindod Wells - the Story of a Spa', with other galleries on archaeology, natural history and social history.

South Glamorgan

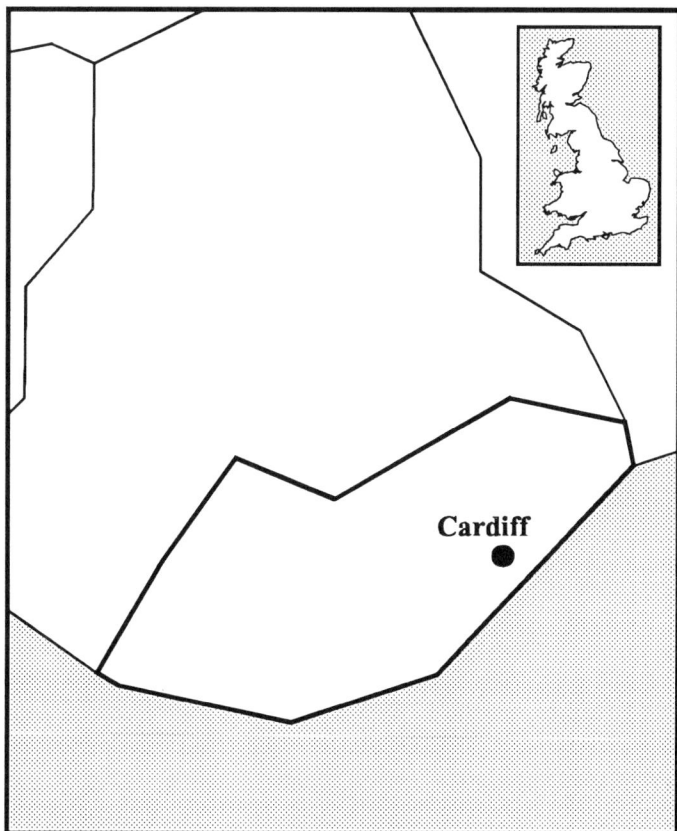

Cardiff
●

WELSH FOLK MUSEUM

ST. FAGANS
CARDIFF CF5 6XB
SOUTH GLAMORGAN

☏ TELEPHONE: 0222-569 441
OPEN: MONDAY - SUNDAY ....10.00 - 5.00
1ST APRIL - 31ST OCTOBER
MONDAY - SATURDAY................................10.00 - 5.00
1ST NOVEMBER - 31ST MARCH
ADMISSION: CHARGE

SHOP. REFRESHMENTS. TOILETS. SPECIAL EVENTS &
TEMPORARY EXHIBITIONS.

  ♿ DISABLED ACCESS TO MOST AREAS.

St. Fagan's Castle and grounds were generously donated
to the National Museum of Wales in 1947 thus enabling the
Folk Museum to be created. This large open-air site of 100
acres is near junction 33 of the M4 motorway.

The indoor galleries house exhibitions showing daily
life, costume and farming implements. In the open-air section
some 30 original buildings from all over Wales have been
moved and carefully re-erected to show how people lived at
various times from 1500 to the present day. Several of the
buildings house the museum's working craftsmen, the corn-
miller, saddler, baker, smith, wood turner, cooper, potter and
weaver.

In the gallery of material culture is a display of medical
instruments including electric treatment apparatus, leech jars,
dental equipment, and artefacts complementing the story of
the famous Welsh general practitioner, chartist and
antiquarian, Dr. William Price, 1800-1893. He was the man
who burnt the body of his son on Llantrisant Common in
1884 and thereby reintroduced cremation to Britain after a
gap of some 1500 years.

Held in store and available by appointment are
amputation sets and other medical items, including a
complete dentist surgery which awaits time and space for
display.

MAIN LIBRARY, CARDIFF UNIVERSITY

UNIVERSITY OF WALES COLLEGE OF MEDICINE
UNIVERSITY HOSPITAL OF WALES
HEATH PARK
CARDIFF CF4 4XN

☏ TELEPHONE: 0222-747 747
    OPEN: .... 10.00 - 5.00
    ADMISSION: FREE

The Library has a large and unique collection of medical books from 1680-1900, including works by Thomas Sydenham, Antonio de Lueeuwenhoek, Herman Boerhaave, Sir John Floyer, Alexander Monro, William Cheselden, William Smellie, William Heberden, Charles Bell, Astley Cooper, Florence Nightingale and reports from various medical societies. These and other works can be seen by serious researchers but a prior appointment must be made.

Appendix A: Blue Plaques in London

ANDERSON, Elizabeth Garrett

1836-1917

20 Upper Berkeley Street
W1

Physician & pioneer of medical
education for women.

ARBUTHNOT, John

1667-1735

11 Cork Street
W1

Scottish physician & wit.

BARNARDO, Thomas John

1845-1905

58 Solent House
Ben Jonson Road
Tower Hamlets

Doctor & founder of homes
for destitute children

BARRIE, Sir James

1860-1937

100 Bayswater Road
Bayswater

Author of Peter Pan whose royalties
go to The Hospital for Sick Children,
Great Ormond St.

BERLIOZ, Hector

1803-1869

58 Queen Anne Street
Westminster

Originally studied medicine until he
was allowed to pursue a career in music.
Stayed here in 1851

BOOTT, Dr. (House)

52 Gower Street
Bloomsbury

The site of the first ether anaesthetic
19th December 1846

BRIGHT, Richard

1789-1858

11 Saville Row
Mayfair

Physician, studied diseases
of the kidney at Guy's.

BUCKLAND, Francis Trevelyan

1826-1880

Surgeon and naturalist

37 Albany Street
Garden of the Royal
College of Physicians

CAVELL, Edith

1865-1915

Pioneer of nursing in Belgium
& heroine of WW1

Nurses Home
London Hospital
Whitechapel

CHADWICK, Sir Edwin

1800-1890

Pioneer of public health

9 Stanhope Terrace
W2

CONAN DOYLE, Sir Arthur

1859-1930

Doctor & author of Sherlock Holmes

12 Tennison Road
South Norwood

DALE, Sir Henry Hallett

1875-1968

Physiologist, Director of National
Institute for Medical Research &
Nobel prize winner 1936

Mount Vernon House
Mount Vernon
Hampstead

DARWIN, Charles

1809-1882

Naturalist, discoverer of
natural selection.

Biological Sciences Building,
Gower Street.

DICK-REID, Dr Grantly

1890-1959

20th Century pioneer of natural
childbirth

25 Harley Street
W1

DRYSDALE, Dr Charles Vickery

1874-1961

Founder of the Family Planning
Association, opened his first
clinic on this site.

153a East Street
Walworth

ELLIS, Henry Havelock

1859-1939

Pioneer in the study of the
Psychology of Sex

14 Dover Mansions
Canterbury Crescent
Lambeth

FLEMING, Sir Alexander

1881-1955

Discoverer of penicillin
also
Laboratory site

20a Danvers Street
Kensington & Chelsea

St. Mary's Hospital

FREUD, Sigmund

1856-1939

Founder of psychonanalysis

20 Maresfield Gardens
Swiss Cottage

GOLDSMITH, Oliver

1728-1774

Doctor, playwright, novelist &
poet

6,Wine Office Court
Temple Church Yard

GRACE, William Gilbert

1848-1915

Cricketer, practised medicine
in Bristol

Fairmount
Mottingham Lane
SE9

GRAY, Henry

1827-1861

Anatomist, author of book
of anatomy

8 Wilton Street
Westminster

GULL, Sir William

1816-1890

Physician at Guy's Hospital
Discoverer of myxoedema

74 Brook Street
Mayfair

HODGKIN, Thomas

1798-1866

Pathologist, described glandular disease

35 Bedford Square
Bloomsbury

HORSLEY, Sir Victor

1857-1916

25 Cavendish Square
W1

Neurosurgeon & physiologist

HOWARD, John

1726-1790

23 Great Ormond Street
WC1

Prison reformer, enforcing
cleanliness

HUNTER, John

1728-1793

31 Golden Square
Soho

Surgeon, anatomist & father
of scientific surgery

HUNTER, William

1718-1783

Lyric Theatre
Great Windmill Street

Anatomist, surgeon-accoucher

HUTCHINSON, Sir Jonathan

1828-1913

15 Cavendish Square
W1

Surgeon, Professor of Surgery
at the Royal London Hospital

HUXLEY, Thomas Henry

1825-1895

38 Marlborough Place
NW8

Biologist, expounder of
Darwin's theories on evolution

JACKSON, John Hughlings

1835-1911

3 Manchester Square
W1

Neurologist

JONES, Ernest

1879-1958

19 York Terrace East
Regents Park

Pioneer Psychonalyst

KEATS, John
1795-1821

Poet & doctor

Keats's House
Wentworth Place
Hampstead

KLEIN, Melanie
1882-1960

Psychoanalyst & pioneer of
child analysis

42 Clifton Hill
NW8

LINACRE, Thomas
1460-1524

Physician, founded Royal
College of Physicians, 1518

Knightrider Street
St. Paul's

LISTER, Joseph, Lord
1827-1912

Surgeon, founder of the
aseptic technique

12 Park Crescent
Regents Park

LITTLE, William John
1810-1894

Physician, founder of Royal
Orthopaedic Hospital

'Red Lion' Aldgate
The City

MACKENZIE, Sir James
1853-1925

Physician, authority on the heart,
invented polygraph to record
its action

17 Bentinck Street
W1

MACKENZIE, Sir Morell
1837-1892

Laryngologist, attended
the German Crown Prince

242 High Road
Leytonstone

MANSON, Sir Patrick
1844-1922

Founder of modern Tropical Medicine,
known as 'Mosquito Manson'

50 Welbeck Street
W1

MARSDEN, William

1796-1867

65 Lincoln's Inn Fields
WC2

Surgeon, founder of the Royal Free
Hospital & Marsden Hospital for
Incurable Diseases

MAUGHAM, William Somerset

1874-1965

6 Chesterfield Street
W1

Novelist & playwright, medical training
at St. Thomas's Hospital

MOORCROFT, William

1767-1825

Littlewoods
Oxford Street

Veterinary surgeon & explorer

NIGHTINGALE, Florence

1820-1910

10 South Street W1
& 90 Harley Street

Established the profession of
nursing which formed the basis
of modern health care

OLIVER, Percy Lane

1878-1944

5 Colyton Road
Southwark

Founder of the first voluntary
blood donor service

PARKINSON, James

1755-1824

1 Hoxton Square
N1

Physician, first described
paralysis agitans

PLACE, Francis

1771-1854

21 Brompton Square
SW3

Political reformer & pioneer
of the study of birth control

PRIESTLEY, Joseph

1733-1804

Ram Place
Hackney
E9

Presbyterian minister & chemist
Discoverer of oxygen

RADCLIFFE, Sir John

1650-1714

19-20 Bow Street
WC2

Physician, bequeathed the bulk of
his fortune to Radcliffe Library,
Infirmary and Observatory, Oxford,
& St Bartholomew's Hospital

RIZAL, Dr Jose

1861-1896

37 Chalcot Crescent
NW1

Philipino patriot & political writer, qualified
in Madrid but executed as a possible
leader of the anti-Spanish revolt on the island

ROBINSON, James

1813-1862

14 Gower Street
Bloomsbury
W1

Pioneer of anaesthesia and dentistry

ROSS, Sir Ronald

1857-1932

18 Cavendish Square
W1

Physician & discoverer of the mosquito
transmission of malaria
Nobel Laureate 1902

SEACOLE, Mary

1805-1881

157 George Street
W1

Jamacian nurse who joined Florence
Nightingale in the Crimea

SIMON, Sir John

1816-1904

40 Kensington Square
Kensington

Pathologist & pioneer of public health
dealing with water supplies and
sewage disposal

SLOANE, Sir Hans

1660-1753

4 Bloomsbury Place
Bloomsbury

Physician, refounded the Chelsea Physic
Garden & leased it to the Society of
Apothecaries.His museum & library formed
nucleus of the British Museum

SMILES, Samuel

1812-1904

11 Granville Park
Lewisham

Surgeon, social reformer
& author of 'Self-Help'

SMOLLETT, Tobias

1721-1771

16 Lawrence Street
Chelsea

Novelist & surgeon

WAKLEY, Thomas

1795-1862

35 Bedford Square
Bloomsbury

Reformer & founder of the *Lancet*

WELLCOME, Sir Henry

1853-1936

6 Gloucester Gate
Regents Park

Pharmacist & founder of Wellcome
Trust, Foundation & Institute for the
History of Medicine

WESLEY, John

1703-1791

47 City Road
EC1

Founder of Methodism & author
of 'Primitive Physick'

WILLAN, Dr Robert

1757-1812

10 Bloomsbury Square
Bloomsbury

Dermatologist & first physician
to classify skin diseases

WILSON, Edward Adrian

1872-1912

Physician, naturalist & explorer
with Scott to Antartica

Battersea Vicarage
42 Vicarage Crscent
Wandsworth

WYNDHAM, Sir Charles

1837-1919

Doctor & actor-manager.
Opened Wyndham's Theatre 1899

19 York Terrace East
W 1

YOUNG, Thomas

1773-1829

Physician, physicist & Egyptologist,
helped decipher the Rosetta Stone
hieroglyphics

48 Welbeck Street
W 1

Appendix B: Statues of Medical People in London

Dr. Thomas John Barnardo

1845-1905   Whitechapel Road

Founder of homes for destitute children
Medical training at the Royal London Hospital

Louisa Aldrich Blake M.D., M.S.

1862-1925   Tavistock Square (South East Corner)

Dean, Royal Free Hospital School of Medicine for Women, 1914 -
1925
Consulting Surgeon, Royal Free Hospital 1919-1925
Surgeon, Elisabeth Garrett Anderson Hospital 1895-1925

Edith Cavell

1865-1915   St. Martin's Place

Nurse trained at Royal London Hospital
Matron of a training school for nurses in Brussels
Helped Belgian and allied servicemen escape
Executed by Germans
*"Patriotism is not enough, I must have no hatred or bitterness
for anyone."*

Thomas Coram

1668-1751   Brunswick Square

Shipwright, philanthropist and founder of the first
institution for ill and destitute children in 1739 - The Foundling
Hospital

Sigmund Freud

1856-1939   Adelaide Road, Swiss Cottage

Austrian founder of psychoanalysis
He spent the last year of his life in Hampstead

Thomas Guy

1644-1724   Courtyard of Guy's Hospital, Southwark

Philanthropist and founder of Guy's Hospital

William Harvey
1578-1657   Museum of Mankind, Burlington Gardens

Physician and discoverer of the circulation of the blood, published
1628

John Hunter
1728-1793   Lincoln's Inn Fields (South West Corner)
& Museum of Mankind, Burlington Gardens
& St. George's Hospital, Tooting
& Leicester Square

Surgeon and physiologist
Founder of scientific surgery

Edward Jenner
1749-1821   Kensington Gardens (West Side)

Physician and discoverer of vaccination against small-pox.

John Keats
1795-1821   Park Lane

Poet and doctor, trained at Guy's Hospital
Qualified at Worshipful Society of Apothecaries.

Joseph Lister
1827-1912   Portland Place

Surgeon and pioneer of the technique of antiseptic surgery

David Livingstone
1913-1873   Royal Geographical Society, Kensington Gore

Doctor and missionary in Central Africa
Died in Africa, buried in Westminster Abbey

John Locke
1632-1704   Museum of Mankind, Burlington Gardens

Physician, philosopher and founder of philosophical liberalism

Sir James McGrigor
Bart M.D., K.C.B., K.C., K.C.T.S., F.R.S.

Atterbury Street, Millbank

Director General of the Army Medical Department 1815-1851
Brought treatment of the wounded into the front line in the
Peninsular War so avoiding the long journeys to the hospital tents

Florence Nightingale
1820-1910

St. Thomas's Hospital
& Waterloo Place

Nurse & hospital reformer

Joseph Priestley
1733-1804

Royal Institute of Chemistry, Russell Square

Presbyterian minister and chemist
He discovered oxygen in 1774

Dr. Alfred Salter
Died 1945

Cherry Gardens, Bermondsy

Bermondsey doctor who was a tireless campaigner for
improvements in public health in working class Bermondsey
from 1900 onwards
Six year old daughter & cat are at the railings overlooking
the Thames

Sir Hans Sloane
1660-1753

Chelsea Physic Garden
& British Museum

Physician & collector
Formed the nucleus of the British Museum

Dr. Bentley Todd
Died 1860

King's College Hospital
Denmark Hill

Anatomical physician and teacher
Founder of King's College Hospital

John Wesley
1703-1791

Wesley's Chapel, City Road

Founder of Methodism
Writer of The Primitive Physic and user of electrotherapy

Index A - Subjects

N

T

U

V

W

X

Index B - Museums

S